WHY BLACK PEOPLE CAN'T LOSE WEIGHT

The Psychology, The Challenge, and The Solution To Overall Wellness

by

Makeisha Lee

authorHOUSE®

AuthorHouse™
1663 Liberty Drive, Suite 200
Bloomington, IN 47403
www.authorhouse.com
Phone: 1-800-839-8640

First published by AuthorHouse 10/31/2007

ISBN: 978-1-4343-4738-1 (sc)

Printed in the United States of America
Bloomington, Indiana

This book is printed on acid-free paper.

Dedication

This book is dedicated to my mother whom I admire, love and respect. Thank you for believing in me and giving me words of encouragement, every step of the way while writing this book.

Thanks mommy and I love you! Much love to all my brothers and my sisters that showered me with love and attention through the years!

This is also dedicated to my grandmother, Mary A. Smith, who struggled with her weight at her heaviest before death (300 pounds) and passed away from complications of stroke and an adverse reaction to prescription medications. She was among an astonishing rate of 2.2 million deaths that result annually from adverse drug reactions. She left this world too soon, and she is sorely missed by the entire family.

This book commemorates the life and death of Russell Lee, my surrogate grandfather and friend whom we lost due to complications of heart disease and obesity. This one is for you; we will see you on the other side!

ACKNOWLEDGEMENTS

This is to acknowledge first and foremost my creator - for without him none of my success in life would be possible. I thank him everyday of my life for giving me the talents, courage, and love within to carry out my purposes and missions in life.

I would also like to acknowledge my dear husband and partner in life Dante Lee, who inspired me to pursue my passion with a sense of purpose and providing technical support every step of the way. Thanks hunny!

Thanks kids: Zahkiyah, Naeem, Cherish, Kylie and DJ for being obedient, cooperative and understanding when mommy had to work and get things done. Love all of you!

Many thanks to all those whom have touched my life in one way or another at some point or another: Eric Campbell, Bertha Jackson, Karen Copeland, Bobbie Copeland, Juanita, Diane Wynona, Gwen, Lisa, Ma. Thanks David Hebb - the male version of myself, and just know that you are on your way up, so stay up!

DISCLAIMER

This book contains only the author's opinions, thoughts and conclusions. It is for educational purposes only and you and only you are responsible if you choose to do anything based on what you read.

The information contained in this book is for educational purposes only. While the author has made every effort to ensure that the content includes accurate and up-to-date information, the author makes no warranties or representations as to the accuracy of the content and assumes no liability or responsibility for any error or omission in the content.

This book does not represent or warrant; that use of any content will not infringe rights of third parties. The author is not affiliated with any medical institution and the content has not been approved by the Food and Drug Administration, the Federal Trade Commission or any other government agency. Neither the author nor the content can be relied upon as preventive, cure, or treatment for any disease or medical condition.

It is recommended that you consult with an appropriate health professional or physician before acting upon any recommendation that is made via the author. Use of this book is at your own risk.

This book is intended as a sharing of knowledge and information from the research and experience of the author in the community.

CONTENTS

A FINAL NOTE TO READERS   149

PRELUDE

Weight loss. Why is it such a vicious cycle? Why does it seem unattainable for us as a community, despite the hundreds of diet plans available? Why do we as Blacks lead in the highest percentage of obesity cases in all gender, age and ethnic groups to date? These questions deserve convincing and satisfying answers.

This book acknowledges that people of African descent could come from of all parts of the earth including from Jamaica, Africa, Canada, Dominican Republic, Brazil, Central America, Europe or elsewhere. Given such, we would simply like to specifically address some unique challenges that "Blacks" encounter on their journey to complete wellness including obesity.

It should be emphasized that when you are "well" you are not obese, as we have come to understand that obesity is a disorder. The two go hand in hand. Of course though, not all thin people are well either; based on the sheer fact that they don't have fat in their body puts them at great risk too with their overall health. This is why understanding how to be well in general is also revealed in this book, making it relevant for all, big and small.

With regards to obesity many of us will allow ourselves to just be swayed by whatever our peers tell us without conducting any research of our own to try to answer some of these questions that come to mind.

We are inundated with T.M.I. (Too Much Information) and every one of us is in a state of information overload.

Being so, it is fully understood that you are not merely looking for more information that has simply been recycled, but rather you want solutions that will give you tangible results at the precise moment that you need it. You want trusted resources that have already sifted through information, filtered it out, leaving only that which is perfect for you in a way that is useful and enjoyable.

In this book, we will answer all the questions you may have had unanswered before; done just so, in a clear concise manner without getting too technical as many other articles, books, and other informational sources often do. This written work of art will reveal all the hidden schemes that mainstream society has kept from us, and break it down so that a 3-year old can understand why we as "Blacks" have been unsuccessful as a whole at getting and/or keeping the weight off.

When you have finished reading this book and taking in all of the insightful, thought-provoking, up close and personal, and in-your-face delivery of information - you will have no doubts about what to avoid and what method you should employ to end this repetitive cycle of obesity and sickness.

You are invited to take off your blinders, put your thinking cap on, let your guard down, and open your mind and heart - as this book was written by one of your own.

It was written with a view to facilitate a rescue of a people who grope for a way out of ill health brought on by obesity. So many other books have been written regarding weight loss, but completely lack cultural sensitivity to African Americans whom need the most attention. When they write their books on what should work for everybody to improve their health, it's like sending the zookeeper in to manage your bank account. Who would rely and trust in that?

 The one illuminative fact that will permeate throughout this entire book is this: We cannot even begin to confront obesity and/or its related illnesses without first addressing the toxicity in our bodies that exists. Obesity cannot ever be completely solved for a single one of us, until toxicity on all levels is under control.

Remember these three facts from Dr. Gus Prosch, M.D. - a leading obesity expert - that will forever change your viewpoints on the disorder of obesity.

1) Anyone can lose weight and keep it off, so long as underlying factors that contribute to obesity and excessive weight gain are determined and properly addressed.

2) Successful weight loss CAN NOT be achieved solely through fad diets, weight loss supplements or an exercise program.

3) It is impossible for those who are obese to eat the same way as "normal" people eat and stay thin.

All things considered, we must go back to the basics and define what obesity is, as certain fundamental issues need to be addressed to arrive at a solution.

In brief, obesity is when one's weight is 20% over recommended maximum weight for one's age and or height. Internally it's when the body is not fully capable of storing proteins and carbohydrates, so excess is converted to fat and stored. Imagine that one pound of fat represents about 3,500 excess calories. So when we don't have the right balance of foods and adequate physical activity, we end up with obesity. According to the Center for Disease Control and Prevention (CDC), 52% of Black women are obese and about 30% of Black men are obese. This is the highest amongst all ethnic groups.

The fad diet industry will always argue over the best approach to losing weight, which is always a high-stake gamble. Realistically, there is virtually no sustainable proof that one fad diet is better than another. This is a huge contributing factor to why weight loss is nothing short of a vicious cycle and a war itself for African Americans (and others) who are trying to lose weight!

Since we as a race account for the largest amount of obese persons in this country, let's address and delve a little deeper. Let's specifically look into the facts surrounding Blacks and obesity, and issues indicative of our community - no longer denying that we have some unique concerns.

We must look at this issue from all perspectives in order to implement a change. We have been told for the last decade that obesity is our own fault. We've been told that obesity is a result of our genetics, but it's not that simple. Before the conclusion of the matter, we all will be better able to understand our challenge in a different light!

Too many lives have been ruined for long enough from misinformation. So without further ado, let's sink our teeth into this life altering, eye-opening information!

1.

THE BREAKDOWN OF OBESITY

Before you pre-judge where this is going, let's get things straight right from the start. This is not intended to blame and negate personal responsibility with respects to our plight. However, certain factors cannot be ignored as being contributory to why progress tends to be an uphill battle, even when personal responsibility is being taken.

When it comes to obesity, we the people of the American society look to the government to guide us in the right direction for solutions. Such can be likened to a person traveling in unfamiliar territory who requires the guidance of a map. That is what a map is - a simplified depiction of a space that highlights objects within that space to help guide you from one point to another.

What would happen if a person (without a good map) went out onto the open road to get to a specific destination that they were only vaguely familiar with? With no appropriate guide to follow, most likely they would get lost and an infinite number of things could and would go wrong. Equally as catastrophic it would be if they had a map, but that map was outdated. Worse yet, suppose the map displayed an incorrect symbol, or omitted a certain key to identify a specific location.

This analogy symbolizes us (the African-American people) being in need of direction, looking to the government to be our compass so that we can use the "map" to get us out of the wilderness of obesity. The map that we are supposed to follow is identified as the USDA's food pyramid. This map has gotten us so far off course that we are at a location in life that is not even on the map!

If anybody had any nagging doubts as to how the Standard American Diet (SAD) regulated by our government got out of hand and got us all going in the wrong direction; this was answered live nationally. An ABC News primetime special corroborated everything those of us in the alternative health field have identified as one of the main culprits of obesity for years.

Peter Jennings, the late news anchor, boldly interviewed members of the food industry. Through their answers to his straight-forward questions, some terrible facts were revealed. It gave everyone the real truth of the history of the role that the food industry has played into the encouragement of obesity in this country.

The interview exposed the fact that the U.S. government and its policies actually promote the act of overeating, which makes it very difficult to fight obesity. We definitely needed this breakdown on the history of the food industry because in order to correct a problem, we must fully understand how the problem really started in the first place. Failure to understand and be aware of all of the not-so-obvious dynamics will cause us to have a crippled recovery.

Recounting the events that led up to this whole epidemic, consider that the government and food industry have American farmers growing and producing more food than we really need. Thus, the more we eat the fatter we get. They also have the agriculture and subsidy connection where Congress will make certain political decisions to provide a higher subsidy for foods that are less nutritious, opposed to foods that are healthier and keep our bodies leaner.

Subsidy is a monetary grant that is paid by the government to a specific group, which in this case, is American farmers. Governments will implement these laws and policies with a goal of achieving a very specific outcome.

Sugars, fats, and dairy get twenty times more subsidy from the government than that of the more healthy foods like fruits and vegetables. Meat and dairy gets three times more subsidy than that of grains. The amount of corn that has been grown and processed has increased three times the amount since the year 1995. Why?

Well, as was highlighted in the Peter Jennings interview, corn is the principle source for sweeteners in American foods. Corn sweeteners are consumed the most out of any other form. It's cheap and you can make almost anything out of it, especially the high calorie foods. It is found in thousands of products we use everyday. This is where agriculture and health policies disconnect. It is no longer important to provide subsidy for the foods that supply good nutrition because funds are allocated to grow the foods that allow them to bring in even more money. From corn they can make sugars, sugar water

3

(beverages), flour, fat and starch - all of which are advocated in the old USDA food pyramid.

The USDA's pyramid was originally designed for the post-war era in 1950 when people were supposedly suffering from malnutrition with diseases such as rickets and lack of vitamin D in their diets. They were thought to be smaller and said to not have been consuming enough calories or enough fat.

Thus, out of this message came the creation of the food pyramid to get everyone to eat more corn, eat more beef, more dairy, and to just eat as much as possible. That is exactly what everyone starting doing.

This proved to be directly for the benefit of the National Dairy Council, The American Meat Institution, The National Cattleman Beef Association and the Wheat Foods Council.

Well into the 80's, 90's, and up until the present we have been following the outdated food guide. However, we are really living in a society that has too much food with no nutrition to support good health.

Only recently in 2007 was this pyramid revised. Sadly, this wasn't done before the health crisis exploded. Unfortunately the updated food pyramid conveniently left out any advice to limit the intake of added sugars. This is because the soft drink companies, sugar industry and mass food producers intensely lobbied against it, citing that there sales would be decreased. The end result - continuity of Diabetes, obesity and other ailments due to the fact that people will inevitably continue to eat those foods, feeling there is no real danger.

The food industry devises deliberate strategies to get people to eat more food while using the cheapest of the cheap food ingredients. These are known as "mass distribution, low-cost products".

Most supermarkets will literally have on the shelves thirty to forty thousand different products that are packaged and processed. This food that is processed allows them to make tons of money because the food ingredients are dirt cheap to make, and the product itself can be sold at a much higher price because they are branded. These food processing companies strip away 98% of the natural nutrition in foods and make huge profits doing so. Processed foods are stripped and refined of all the good elements like wheat, fiber and essential oils. By the time they are done refining everything, nothing of real nutritional value is left.

Then they proceed to douse us everywhere we go with free samples of pudding, cakes, cookies, chips, pies, etc. And we eat it all up because it tastes good, as these foods are higher on the glycemic index. This simply means that the moment you put it into your mouth even before you swallow, it breaks down into sugar instantly. People generally feel the narcotic-like effect right away. They (the food industry) go to great lengths to make sure that this stuff taste so good so that you cannot resist.

If you want to know if these tactics are working on us (Blacks) in particular, consider this: According to Target Market News, black households spend approximately two billion dollars a year purchasing cookies, cakes, pies and so forth.

Did you know that Kraft Foods® which is owned by Phillip Morris® (a cigarette company) has thousands of employees working around the clock just reorganizing molecules in food to make you want to continue to buy these foods? Companies like them make it their business to know and construct ways to entice and tantalize your taste buds - essentially transforming you into an addict. Why else would they need such a rigorous intelligence force allocated?

Kraft's very own food study that was conducted on African American consumers indicated that Blacks eat junk food snacks more often with a preference for odd combinations such as salty and sweet. Through their study, they are also able to determine precisely what motivates us to purchase certain foods, and then they are more than happy to oblige us.

They have figured out that we are motivated to buy brand name versus private label because of the misconception that we will be getting a better quality of food. This couldn't be further from the truth! As was pointed out earlier - the larger the company, the more chemicals they will use in the processing of their foods; the cheaper the ingredients equals greater profits. When we are addicted to their foods, we become their loyal customer base. There are some very specific chemicals they use to accomplish their goal of keeping us addicted that you will find out about as you read on.

Basically, here you are - unsuspecting, thinking that it's your entire fault and that you have no willpower whatsoever. Picture that scenario of people conducting their own food psychoanalysis whereby they deliberately alter food to taste abnormally scrumptious and then studying how we react like we are a bunch of lab rats.

How does untainted, healthy nutritious food compete with food that has not been enhanced in any way? People's taste buds are so whacked out nowadays that clean, fresh, organic, natural foods do not taste good to them, instead we are accustomed to eating processed foods. Some express that they don't want natural or organic because it tastes bland. Some don't even crave foods that are chemical-free, unrefined, or non-GMO (Genetically Modified) in any way. For the record, chemical- free foods ARE tasty and naturally robust with flavor. On the other hand, chemicals may be potent, but find out what else they are, how they are being used, and the effects that they are having on us.

The Truth about NutraSweet, Equal, Trans Fats, and MSG

These substances are found in almost every food product sold in markets, independently or combined. But what exactly are they and why are they considered to be deadly?

Aspartame is marketed as NutraSweet, Equal, and Spoonful and often promoted on labels as sugar-free. Back in 1983, the FDA approved NutraSweet in soft drinks and other liquids and immediately the Center for Disease Control (CDC) and FDA started to receive unprecedented amounts of complaints from people experiencing horrible health issues. There were complaints of depression, hypertension, dementia, nausea, headaches, dizziness, etc.

Leading research proves this artificial sweetener is in fact a poison. When aspartame is stored for long periods of time or in warm areas

- it changes to methanol. Methanol is an alcohol that converts to formaldehyde or formic acid.

Formic acid is the poison found in the sting of fire ants and is a known Carcinogen (cancer-causing agent). No wonder you can be subjected to symptoms of numbness in your lungs, blurred vision, vertigo and even more symptoms upon continuous consumption of aspartame.

We will talk more about the role that the diet industry plays a little later, but it's important for you to be aware that diet products use aspartame and claim that it's good to help you lose weight. The exact opposite is true! These chemically-altered products make you crave carbohydrates so that when you are eating those diet foods or drinking their meal replacement drinks; you will no doubt gain weight. Why so? They all contain aspartame, and the poison in aspartame finds a safe haven in the fat cells.

It is scientifically proven that acid gets stored in fat cells and ultimately creates an acidic environment throughout your body. So the longer you stay acidic the longer you keep fat cells. Next, they become cold due to lack of oxygen - which blocks fuel necessary to burn fat. Once acid is stored, the fat cells need to dilute the poison by retaining fluid. A disaster is just waiting to happen!

What about trans-fats or hydrogenated oils? These are very unhealthy oils that are extremely toxic. There is enough information to conclude that in the long term, consumption of them leads to cardiovascular disease, as they clog the arteries and increase cholesterol levels. The atmosphere they create also encourages strokes and sometimes causes irreparable damage to the nervous system.

Furthermore, there are is an interesting fact that researchers at Wake Forest University uncovered. By conducting a 6-year study on 51 male monkeys, they showed that trans fats largely contribute to dangerous belly fat. In one group, monkeys were given 8% of calories from trans fats and the other given 8% of healthy fats (olive oil). By the end of the study, the monkeys that were fed trans fats had a 7.2% body fat increase and the other 1.8%. The monkeys fed trans fats had a 30% increase in abdominal fat with more body fat from other parts of the body re-distributed to the belly area!

What you want to be concerned about is that these toxic chemical substances are creating an unhealthy environment in our bodies that directly causes imbalances and disorders like obesity. They are still on the market and sometimes ingeniously disguised. DO NOT BE MISLED. All of these are making us fat and giving us disease, yet most of us don't even know it. Be on guard! Trans fats/hydrogenated oils are secretly being added into vitamins used as fillers by vitamin companies to cut cost.

Good news! According to the Center for Media and Democracy (CMD), in July 2007, there was a ban on the use of trans fats in restaurants in New York City passed by the Board of Health.

Mayor Bloomberg states that the Health Department estimates hundreds of lives could be saved annually. In light of this, it is strongly advisable that you eliminate these chemical substances from your diet NOW.

Alternatives for unhealthy oils are: olive oil, un-refined virgin coconut oil, and flax oil.

Alternatives for aspartame and ALL artificial sweeteners including Splenda are: stevia, an all natural herb; and xylitol, equivalent to sugar but has 40% less calories and is absorbed in the blood less slowly making it safe even for diabetics.

An additional benefit to using xylitol for the entire family is this: in 11 clinical trials xylitol was shown to reduce ear infections and cavities in children by 80%. In Sweden, "it's used as chewing gum for preschoolers," says science researcher Dr. Bill Wheeler.

Other natural sweeteners include: date sugar and Agave syrup.

Everyone is encouraged to be prepared for Genetically Engineered Sugar that is scheduled to hit stores in 2008. This sugar is chemically processed from sugar beets that have been modified and sprayed with large amounts of herbicides that contaminate the soil and water.

Now, would be a good time to wake up to the fact that today's society distorts and twists scientific truths of health, nutrition and dietary choices during unethical political processes. These food companies and the USDA are blood buddies. All types of schemes and corruptive practices are on the rise. Why refer to them as such? The USDA with its revision of the food pyramid had THE golden opportunity to inform the public about the damaging effects of the intake of various foods containing harmful substances, such as the latter. They failed once again to enforce education to the public about the good carbohydrates vs. the bad carbohydrates along with good vs. bad fats. Instead, they choose to protect the industry (food companies) and not the consumer. No gumption to stand up and say: "Enough is enough!"

The saying has been, "If you don't know, you better ask somebody." Not in this case though. Chances are, nobody you know has a clue. You thought you knew, but you really didn't - until now. For the skeptics that can't handle the truth, you may conduct your own research and read up on it in a book called *Food Politics* by Marion Nestle, PhD, MPH.

The food industry spends 33 billion dollars each year marketing to the public to encourage eating these foods. They encourage eating larger portions, and tell you that you don't have to change your eating habits if you exercise.

That is a terrible misconception because you have to jog for 15 minutes just to burn 1 oz of a bag of potato chips, and you have to walk for 6 hours just to burn off the calories from a McDonald's combo meal. These companies know that some of us don't buy into the lie, so they will pay health organizations to tell you that you can eat from these places and make it a part of a healthy diet. This is not true at all and the evidence of the effects these foods have on the body prove otherwise. If you drink soda (pop), think about this: you have to ride your bike for an entire hour just to burn off the calories from one can. Plus, it takes the body 17 hours to neutralize the acid in your blood from it.

We have indeed been misled into thinking that various foods are safe to consume on a regular basis. Just because the labels have the words "fresh" or "natural" plastered on them, doesn't mean they are healthy for you. The truth is that these chemicals are deliberately being placed in our foods and are directly causing us to be obese and very sick. Along with NutraSweet, Aspartame, Splenda, and Trans Fats, there is MSG or Monosodium Glutamate.

MSG is a very popular flavor enhancer in many foods (foreign and American). Some manufacturers place "No MSG Added" labels on their products, and the average person will assume that this is safe. However, the reality is that these companies are still hiding MSG in their foods by calling it a different name.

It's a crying shame that we can't simply rely on just reading the labels on the back to determine what and if any harmful substances exist within the product. Rather, we have to play Inspector Gadget and decode the listings because of the misrepresentation on the part of the food industry.

For instance, when referring to soy sauce and other processed flavor enhancers that already contain MSG, the label might read "Hydrolyzed Protein" and/or "Glutamic Acid" or "spices". By listing these ingredients, it is legally acceptable for these companies to make the claim of no added MSG in a given product. They get really clever by adding MSG in (yeast extract) and changing the serving sizes. They know it's in there, but you don't!

But why be concerned?

Well, the food industry continues to make billions at the expense of our health. The use of MSG in food has been directly linked to obesity and countless illnesses. The first researcher to find evidence of such was Dr. John Olney of the Washington University Medical School in St. Louis, MO. In 1968, he found that MSG injected in mice resulted in serious brain damage and obesity. Since then,

MSG has been found to produce the same effect on humans. Dr Russell Blaylock, a retired Neurosurgeon gives informative scientific evidence documenting the actual cell degeneration in brain cells caused by chemical additives.

Are you starting to see a pattern in relations to these chemicals in food that add to the obesity epidemic? With all the fanfare about it; this is not what we are hearing about as causes for obesity, but it's true.

The authors of the published book entitled *The Slow Poisoning of America* found evidence that MSG is in fact very addictive, thus contributing to weight gain. The FDA even admits that MSG has been proven to induce asthma attacks. (Blacks happen to have the highest incidence of death rates from asthma). Hence, we still have the less than amusing, hide and go seek cover-up games with "MSG Replacers" being manufactured as we speak. They hide what's really inside; you have to find out where.

Evidently MSG is so dangerous that other parts of the world have outlawed any and everything that looks like MSG, and they are not doing so just because of its connection to obesity and other ailments, but they also found that the connection between MSG and depression is extremely strong.

It's no secret that processed Chinese food is higher in MSG than even our American food. An article in the BBC in the UK states this about the public health crisis in China: 250,000 people commit suicide each year. Basically, China alone makes up 42% of all suicides committed in the world. These facts were reported by The Hindu – one of India's national newspapers.

What about the implications for us since the introduction of MSG? In between the years 1980-1996, the rate for suicide has increased by 105% in African American males aged 15-19. This was reported by the Center for Disease Control and Prevention (CDC).

Draw your own conclusions based on facts surrounding this issue, but know that one should strive to be safe – rather than sorry.

The chemical additives that have evolved have been produced by a company called Senomyxs. In a recent New York Times article, the CEO of Senomyxs was quoted as saying, "We're helping companies clean up their labels." This deceit is precisely what we as consumers need to watch out for.

This is all designed to keep us physically addicted to the foods, so that we can keep buying and they can keep making money.

A recent European study conducted at the University of Liverpool, concluded that MSG and aspartame in combination with food colorings cause even more harm to nerve cells, than each of the additives alone. This was later published in the Journal of Toxicological Sciences. Despite these findings, the FDA does not acknowledge that adding these substances to our food poses a grave risk to our health. So what does this mean to us?

It means that we have to take the initiative and become aware of the importance of healthy nutrition. We must at all cost avoid foods that have been manipulated and transformed to imitate natural flavors, colors (added for attractiveness), and preservatives. They only add that color to meat to make you think that it is fresh. The color that is typically used is a known carcinogenic called sodium nitrite (nitrates).

A carcinogenic is a cancer-causing agent. At local supermarkets, you can find this chemical in the following products: hot dogs, lunch meats, bacon, and more. Really if you were to see the meat without the red color added in, you would not want to buy it at all!

Read your labels, paying particular attention to the terms "artificial flavoring or coloring" because MSG is being grouped under that labeling.

FOODS WITH MSG

- ✓ Many restaurant soups
- ✓ Most sausages sold at supermarkets
- ✓ Most McDonald's foods (including the salads)
- ✓ KFC fried chicken and most of their products
- ✓ Doritos and Pringles
- ✓ Accent (the spice)
- ✓ Medications in gelcaps (which have glutamic acid in the gelatin)

- ✓ Kraft's products (most contain free glutamate)
- ✓ Gravy Master
- ✓ Marmite
- ✓ Flavored Ramen Noodles
- ✓ Boullon - any kind
- ✓ Flavored potato chips
- ✓ Processed cheese spread
- ✓ Instant soup mixes

For the complete list, visit http://www.msgtruth.org/avoid.htm

Definitely, we want to be more conscious of the need to consume only products that are free from chemicals and additives. When in doubt, do without. 50 million organic consumers are already doing this!

Whatever you eat and/or drink today - walks and talks tomorrow!

Our Youth - How Are They Affected?

Because of the way that the food industry markets to children with the various types of foods, the cultural norm has been changed. When we allow our children to watch television for recreational purposes, they are exposed to a bunch of commercials on what to eat. The average child is subject to 10,000 food ads each year on TV alone, and is encouraged to consume sugar-coated cereal, sugary beverages of all kinds with artificial colorings, and high-fat, salty snacks. The food industry representatives will admit their guilt in the way they market to children. Their explanation is that they do so because they know they won't get the same return promoting healthy foods as much as they would on sugary snacks.

This is all pure insanity because back in the 60's and 70's, our children preferred to eat healthy snacks like fresh fruits. No wonder African American children are becoming more obese than ever before at much younger ages.

There is an alarming concern that we all should have due to the increasing numbers of obese children in our community. Its one matter when we are discussing what used to be a primarily adult issue of obesity; yet quite another when it comes to our youth. This is a very serious issue that we cannot afford to take lightly. The

American Obesity Association reports that 30% of kids ages 6-11 are overweight and 15% are obese.

Even more astounding than that is our children are manifesting some very serious illnesses, like hypertension, diabetes, asthma and sleep apnea. They are not even out of elementary school before they are on their way to a diabetic coma with an inhaler pump in their hands. To that end, they are saying sleep apnea in children in fact may be even more prevalent in African Americans because obesity, a strong risk factor, tends to be more common in this group.

This is disturbing since the numbers have increased by more than 120% among African Americans as compared to 50 percent among whites within a decade. So the question is, if they are suffering with these serious health challenges as a direct result from obesity at age 11, will they be around to see 30, 40 or 20 even? Likely if this continues, our very own youth will be the first in the nation's history not to live longer than their parents.

We all know that with these little mini-markets on every corner of the neighborhood, children don't have to go very far to have unlimited access to these unhealthy foods. Their strategy for keeping us fat is simple multiplication: make it easy and convenient to get these foods (x) times, encouraging eating larger portions (x) times encouraging eating more frequently = obesity.

If that is unachievable for whatever reason, the schools certainly will get in on the money bandwagon with promotion of vending machines in the schools. Many parents are unaware that these schools earn revenues through soda and candy manufacturers by allowing the sales of these snacks via the vending machines.

Target Market News estimates that Black households spend almost 3 times more money annually on meals from vending machines and in school cafeterias than their white counterparts. Ninety percent of the food being introduced via school lunch programs to our kids is pure "junk". This fact of serving up high calorie, caffeine and sugar-laced, low nutritious food along with limited or activity is having a devastating effect. Children are not active enough during the day because a lot of the required physical education programs are being cut out. They are doing this in other communities, but where do you think they make the cuts first?

Ann Cooper, author of *Lunch Lessons - Changing The Way We Feed our Children* states that 78% of schools in America do not actually meet USDA's nutritional guidelines. That's scary considering that we know the standards of the USDA are not high enough with regard to proper nutrition to begin with. Ann Cooper also noted that most food service systems have completely retreated from cooking and instead 100% of the food arrives in plastic and is later reheated to serve to the children.

This explosion of childhood obesity has burst on the scene with a fearsome vengeance because of these various tactics employed by professional predators. Our youth are "munching their way to the morgue" while the schools salute them!

Researchers at the Harvard school of public health have conducted studies showing an increase in consumption of soda and sugar-sweetened beverages. They were able to determine its precise impact on children's body weight. Their findings over the course of the study monitored soda, Hawaiian Punch, lemonade, Kool-Aid and other sweetened fruit drinks as well as iced tea; all of which are culprits of obesity. Yet this is what children think they should have and deserve to have, because it's "normal".

Parents we need to take this obesity situation very seriously. If we continue to allow such foods to be the main source of our children's diet, we are participating in and stand guilty as charged in a horrific new form of child abuse! We may be able to handle a charge of D.U.I. (Driving Under Influence), getting away with little more than a monetary price to pay on our record, but none of us are prepared to catch a charge of "D.W.Y." (Dying While Young) on our conscience.

Rather, we should stand up and assert our power in protecting our most valuable asset. Children are gifts from God that we are instructed to care for. Definitely we don't want to be held blood guilty by not taking action.

We may take immediate action to help put an end to this developing trend in our community by giving them nutritious meals before sending them off to school. This will prevent their bodies from going into starvation mode, making them more prone to eat junk.

Here are some tips:

- Have them pack a lunch from home.

- Instead of giving them sweets or candies, don't bring them into the house at all.

- Replace the refrigerator with fresh organic fruits and vegetables. Hungry children will eat what ever is in the home.

- Have eating a moderate portion of sweets as part of special occasions.

- Introduce to their diet daily super foods.

There are some amazing super foods in powder form that contain all the vital fruits and veggies in proper proportions for their growing bodies for your convenience.

Why consider super foods? The fact of the matter is that we don't get enough nutrition in the regular foods we buy from the grocery store. Due to the degradation of the soil in which our food is grown in, it is absolutely necessary to supplement the children's diet as well as our own. For example, an orange contains 40% less vitamin C than it did back in the 60's.

It is true that since we lead very hurried lives, most of us will turn to the quick fixes, processed packaged foods and the like. So, super foods can provide everyone with healthy alternatives that can give exactly the proper servings of foods without sacrificing good nutrition.

Secondly, the consumption of too much cooked foods puts enormous stress on internal organs because natural enzymes are lost during cooking from high temperatures. High temperature is defined as heat over 100 degrees fahrenheit. Superfoods, on the other hand, allow all nutrients to be absorbed directly into the bloodstream.

Whatever you do, you should not put children on a diet, as this could interfere with proper growth development.

As for exercise:

- Let them play a sport or extra curricular activity.

- Take advantage of some of the amazing non-profit organizations nationally and locally trying to educate the entire family on how to incorporate proper physical activity in their daily routine. GET THEM INVOLVED!

- Be a role model for the children. They do as we do, not as we say!

Now that we have acknowledged that there are some other more subtle dynamics at work, we can better equip ourselves on how to bolster our own suit of armor in battling against the bulge. There is yet another arena that serves to take advantage of us when it comes to obesity in our community. That is the fad diet industry. What role does that industry play?

Diet Schemes and Medical Procedures

Cousin James, Aunt Sally, you name it - is on a new diet; Mothers, fathers, doctors, lawyers, college students, and the list goes on. In fact, 91% of female college students have attempted to control weight gain through dieting since they all tend to gain an average of 5-20 pounds between their 1st and 2nd year of college. Does dieting help at all?

Diets, plain and simple, don't work as a permanent solution for weight loss. Diets work *against* your natural biochemistry and program your body to store fat - not release it.

Many diet plans out there that offer meal replacements, use the same cheap ingredients in their foods as do the supermarkets. For instance, NutriSystem® uses ground corn, sugar corn oil, corn syrup solids, modified food starch, and artificial colors (blue #2 and red #40). Their products contain hydrolyzed protein (a common disguise for MSG), and also hydrogenated soybean oil (often disguised as trans-fats). As discussed previously and factually proven, these are harsh chemicals that damage the body.

About fifteen years ago, well-known actor and comedian Sinbad spoke of his brief stint on a NutriSystem® diet program in one of his stand-ups. Not only did he mention that he was always hungry, but he joked about his uncontrollable cravings. Needless to say it was not something he felt worked for him, or even worth the money that he spent on it. While the audience enjoyed the jokes about dieting and getting "had" by these diet schemes, just fast forward 10 years and today it is no laughing matter. They scheme their way into the pockets of obese people in order to make their own pockets fatter.

Companies like NutriSystem® are largely incorporated, which means that they too mass distribute low-cost products. Their foods are highly processed and laden with some 3,000 chemicals that give the foods flavor, color and a longer shelf life. Their packaging also has some 12,000 chemicals.

These factors alone for weight loss systems can cause your body to go out of balance, by your organs becoming bombarded with the build up of toxins. This leads to the system getting clogged, and confused. In an effort to protect itself from these harmful substances, the body will incase the organs in fat and mucus. These will become embedded in the tissues. All of the preservatives in those diet foods make the body work overtime to try and digest.

The truth is though that in most cases, all of the food never even gets digested completely. Instead it sits in the colon, becomes rotten, and over time gets compacted in the intestinal walls of the colon (the body's sewer system) which by now has malfunctioned. The average person has anywhere from 3-15 lbs of undigested fecal matter that slows metabolism down to a snail's pace. The metabolism needs to be completely balanced in order to burn fat efficiently. As the great Stan Watkins would say, "What a mess!"

These diet plans that are supposed to help you burn fat and ultimately lose weight actually cause you to store fat.

Here is the part where you counteract by reasoning that there are diet plans that exist that do in fact help you lose weight. This is true. Most dieters can lose about 10% of their total body weight. However, statistics show that 67% of these dieters regain their body weight within a year after stopping. Then about 95% regain after 5 years, and 33% end up gaining more weight than what they had before they started. This is your typical yo-yo effect that fuels this vicious weight loss cycle.

Here are some important points to remember:

- Diets do not work because they do not address the underlying imbalances in the body and lifestyle factors that are the primary causes of our obesity.

- Diets typically cause imbalances such as that of electrolytes (potassium) and most importantly - nutrients.

Let's consider the myths behind low-fat diets, low-carb diets, and low-calorie diets:

Low-Fat Diets

Being on a low fat diet may help you lose weight, but that is only the beginning of the END. We all, at one time or another, may have attempted to lower our fat intake; perhaps upon the advice of a doctor. We go shopping to get the right foods to help us live up to the low fat diet requirements of either "no fat", or "low fat". What we are offered in these stores are once again processed foods that contribute to obesity. Some of these include: fat free chips, processed fat free cookies, processed fat free ice-cream, and the list goes on. Yet these well-meaning (some) medical doctors within our community in an effort to help overweight African Americans have preached utilizing fat free foods as a form of dieting in their books.

They also promote the use of diet sodas that have aspartame in them. What they don't even bother to tell you is that the carbonation in the soda blocks calcium absorption. They give some the same old advice of exercising, and eating a well-balanced meal three times a day. They claim that this is all you need to stay healthy. That is simply not the case and quite frankly not working well enough. While the exercising is certainly part of the equation, more education on nutritious meals should be emphasized heavily, even insisted.

It is as plain as day to see that; low-fat dieting is a scandalous attempt to increase the sales for the diet industry to further send profits through the roof. Where do they put these kinds of products? Everywhere, making sure that every little corner store in the neighborhood sells these trash foods for your convenience.

This strategy was designed to deliberately make you fat because processed fat-free, or low fat foods, don't really have any real nutrition in them and practically no fiber. As you frequent these stores and purchase these foods with the intent that you are doing a good thing for your body and cut out the fat, your efforts are for naught.

We don't realize that when we eat these foods, the acids in the stomach begin to dissolve the foods and digest them too fast. You are not satisfied and nourished properly from these foods, so you eat more just to get the sensation of fullness. This ripple effect contributes to why the average American has stretched their stomach two to three times its normal size. Internally what happens in the body is that since, processed low-fat foods are loaded with chemicals, these chemicals actually lower your blood sugar levels making you hungry all over again. The repetitive cycle is that you eat more of the processed foods, you take in excess empty calories, and your body stores the extra calories as fat - exactly what you are trying to stay away from.

With the heavy promotion of "low-fat diets", most people are convinced that fat of any kind is taboo. This is the ultimate brainwashing technique. Just doing minimal research on nutrition will prove that healthy fats are not the villain, but can be your best friend when it comes to decreasing body fat.

Numerous vitamins such as A, D, E & K don't even work without good fats. According to the Wholefood Farmacy -whole foods like nuts and seeds contain certain essential fatty acids that your body requires in order to be healthy. The Wholefood Farmacy, based in Rogersville, TN, is a leading supplier of whole food based meals & snacks and is a wonderful alternative to largely incorporated supermarkets. For clarification, "whole" means that the food is still intact and un-manipulated by processing. For instance, if you buy a loaf of wheat bread, the label should read "whole wheat bread". Besides that, whole foods contain fiber. Additionally, fruits, vegetables, nuts, seeds, grains and berries all have good fiber in them.

The acids in your stomach will not completely dissolve these natural fibers, so eating them fills you up quicker and keeps you full longer. One other downside to eating these foods is that these same processed foods contain extra amounts of omega-6 oils which cancel out the body's use of the healthy omega-3 oils. To prevent this we all should be fortifying our bodies with a healthy balance of all three omegas: 3, 6 and 9.

As a recap: The only taboo fats are trans fats, partially hydrogenated oils and excess amounts of animal fats commonly found in fast foods, junk foods, and even diet foods.

It does not matter what the diet plan advertises about as to why it is guaranteed to work; don't believe the hype! It's all part of a greater conspiracy that they think we're easy targets for. All the food and diet industry really care about is making money. They don't care that people buy into their gimmicks out of disparity, or that what they get caught up in is a never-ending cycle of dieting. How many people do you know including yourself have experienced long-term weight loss success?

These "Mickey Mouse" corporation antics are a joke! They are not for real people who want real, lasting results.

People will try one program after another and perhaps lose a few pounds here and there, or even maybe a substantial amount of weight. However, this yo-yo effect with weight over time causes progressive increases in percentage of body fat. Medical studies prove that this composition change is a result of losing lean muscle mass during the diet phase and adding extra fat as the weight is put back on over time.

Low-Carb Diets

Most people who favor this form of dieting have bought into the true meaning of fad, what's new and what's "in". Perhaps from the advice of another professional dieter, they may decide to try their hand at low-carb dieting. Of course the friend made it sound so easy to do by giving them a list of "yes" and "no" foods. Much the same as if you tell one person a certain thing and they tell another, so on and so on. By the time it comes back, it's no where near the same message. So too goes the instructions on the low-carb diet. Most only come away with practicing the portion that tells them all the foods on the "yes" list. They get excited and start eating away; not realizing that over consumption of some of those approved foods can raise the LDL levels - bad cholesterol. They are not aware that the ideal consumption of calories for weight loss is less than 1600 calories a day. A word to the wise: cutting out any food group altogether can be very dangerous and even counterproductive.

The human brain needs 130 grams of carbohydrates per day to function properly. When you opt to only cut out carbohydrates from your diet, you force your body into a diabetic-like state. Your body is quite intelligent and equipped with various survival mechanisms. In this case it knows you need carbohydrates. So it signals danger to the brain and body by responding with very intense cravings that are almost impossible to resist. This is why individuals have been known to experience extreme irritability form low carb dieting. Moreover, it's been said that Dr. Atkins, the founder of the Atkins™ diet was found to be clinically obese, thus causing further investigation into the dangers of this type of dieting.

Ponder over these few facts the next time you think about trying a diet program that promotes low-carbs for weight loss:

- You put yourself at risk for conditions of extreme constipation and/or damage to vital organs such as the kidneys, and liver.

- You may suffer from extreme exhaustion and fatigue.

- Heart disease may be exacerbated or even stroke can occur.

- Fruits are a part of the building blocks of good health and you would be depriving yourself of them while following the low carb diet.

Low-Calorie Diets

This is probably the closest solution to addressing weight issues for individuals, but not without its consequences as well. Calorie restriction can help you lose weight rather quickly, but it too can trigger one of the body's survival mechanisms - which is to store calories in the form of fat. This, in turn could set you up for another disorder of binge eating. So now you have even more challenges to deal with. With calorie restriction the metabolism slows - down, fat cells blow – up and then fatty toxins are stored in the body's tissues. Thus, weight is put back on over time.

Weight Watchers® is a well-known company that promotes low-calorie diets. The danger from calorie restriction can get ugly when a really obese person decides to reduce calories. He or she will lose his normal fat reserves, and once those have been exhausted they will begin to burn structural fat. Here is the real catch: Only as a last resort will the person's body attempt to burn the "abnormal" fats.

Before the person can achieve burning of the abnormal fats, they start to feel so weak and hungry that they wind up quitting the diet. This is the reason why generally people that use this method of dieting feel they look sick; they lost the wrong fat while dieting.

In most cases, they are literally starved and it shows in their faces. We have all seen this look in someone who is fresh off a diet; hunger gives their faces a sunken look. They are smaller, but there belly, hips, thighs and upper-arms have barely improved. They might even have a lot of loose skin too.

Severe calorie restriction can be especially unpleasant and dangerous if you (like most obese people) have other health problems such as heart disease or diabetes.

So if calorie restriction is your choice of dieting, it should be done in balance and in proportion to your individual BMI (Body Mass Index) to avoid the above effects.

Another important factor is cost. These diets that have weight loss centers are more expensive than you might calculate or anticipate. They have you attend meetings for a price, and of course you have to pay for their pre-packaged meals; which is nothing more than packaged fast-foods. Nonetheless, they can be given one point for the group support which can be very helpful for those that have the time to attend. *Weight watchers members know what this means.*

Magic Weight Loss Pill Scams and More Diet Schemes

How many of us have been ripped off by one of those advertisements for instant weight loss? You know how it reads: "Lose 20 lbs. in 5 days. Get rid of that stubborn belly fat. Never work out again and lose 50 lbs. Get thin, slim and trim, just take one pill a day." Akavar's diet slogan is "Eat all you want and still lose weight." It's all scams. They prey on the desperate and also people that are less educated about their deceptive tactics. In many cases, this describes African American people.

There are thousands of such companies within the diet industry promoting these magic potions and pills as a permanent solution to weight loss. They also will make misleading claims about the potency, quality and quantity of their products. Just take a look at the most recent and largest weight loss pill scam to hit North America: The Pure Hoodia, Inc.

Health investigations published by *Truth Publishing Inc.* revealed that Hoodia Gordonii™ is no miracle weight loss pill at all, and that two-thirds of Hoodia pills sold in the US are counterfeit. Pure Hoodia, Inc. operates several companies which are advertised and promoted as separate companies, but are actually owned and controlled by the same people. These are huge implications because how do you actually know what diet pill is tied into this scam? Or, what other weight loss pill companies may be doing the same thing?

Then there's Cortislim™ - the pill out that guarantees you can get rid of abdominal fat without liposuction. The truth is that Cortislim™ puts caffeine in their products, which actually activates cortisol (a stress hormone) into your body. Caffeine also causes your body to store fat. Any substance that contains harsh stimulants can get weight off, but what is it doing to your health? We will find out exactly what it has been doing to our health when we discuss the chronic disease burden for Blacks in the coming chapters.

This type of pill and many others say things like - "Lose the flab in hours with no work." Don't buy into that hype. To begin with, if you really want to get rid of abdominal fat, you're going to have to take an "all over" approach. This is done by decreasing body fat overall. It is biologically and mathematically impossible to lose abdominal fat alone, particularly without consistent physical activity. Fat will not just magically disappear from one particular place on the body just because you rubbed something on, or you popped a wonder pill. Here are some facts to consider:

1) Your body ultimately is the determining factor on where the fat will go and how it will be removed. The credit for this goes to something we all have – genetics.

2) Due to biomechanics, the midsection or abdominal area of your body is the best place to store extra energy in the form of fat.

3) Doing hundreds of crunches or eating certain foods, and taking certain herbs and potions alone is not going to remove fat from the belly, opposed to another body part. There are fat cells all over the body.

4) Males tend to lose body fat in this order: first, it will come off your face, then arms and legs. Next, it will come off your upper body then the buttocks, and a man should not allow his midsection to go over 40".

5) Women will tend to lose fat on the buttocks and hips last. For both males and females, abdominal fat is generally the last fat to get rid of. A woman should not allow her midsection to exceed 35".

Some might say that they would never buy those over-the-counter weight loss pills, but would trust a prescribed weight loss pill that is FDA approved. A good example is the Phen Phen that was FDA approved, and claimed so many lives. Well, there are still others out there on the market right now, some 100 new ones in the process of being approved as you read this information. These DRUGS can cause increased heart rate and heart rhythm irregularities and stroke. No matter what the marketers say about these diet drugs and pills they are not good for you at all and should not be used for long term weight loss.

They may tell you that this pill can "block fat" so your body cannot absorb it, like the ALLI™ diet. That is the line they are running. After all, you might think that it's working because you can actually see the fat in your oily stool. Although that's the case, being on this diet pill will interfere with the absorption of good fats and fat soluble vitamins.

While ALLI™ promoters are currently using everyone as human guinea pigs, we will have to sit back and wait in similar fashion to the Phen Phen deal to see what effects it will have on the body. There is currently no safety data on the use of this drug beyond two years! If you decide to participate in this experimental process - proceed with caution and rest assured that the outcome will prove to be the same for all professional dieters: FAILURE!

What about the topical gels? Some may rationalize that it's not a diet, or a pill so it should be safe enough to use for weight loss. Wrong again!

Topical cutting gels, such as Dermalin, give a temporary and limited amount of results, but the manufacturers clearly state in their application instructions that the fat may be redistributed or end up in other parts of the body. How nutty is that? If fat is going to be redistributed in the body, you may as well have kept it where it was in the first place; either on the hips, abdomen, thighs or where ever. Besides that, since they are highly toxic fat solvents - people who want to get healthy and stay healthy should never use these.

This is not what the weight loss and diet pill companies will tell you, of course. Why would they? But it is the truth. Make no mistake about it; obesity *is* the most pressing public health crisis since tobacco smoking, which claims so many lives. We, being overweight African Americans, are facing the same outcome and it's not a matter of "if", it's "when"!

If you haven't been "had" by any of those trends and forms of dieting, surely you may have tried and or contemplated some of the latest most popular diets. The lemonade diet has spread quicker than a southern California forest fire. This one has every woman thinking she is going to look like Beyonce, the superstar who endorsed the diet. While it may provide some great health benefits along with initial weight loss, will the average person be able to easily integrate this diet plan into their everyday life?   There is no way that a diet of only four ingredients (maple syrup, lemon, cayenne and sea salt) has the capabilities of sustaining life in the healthiest way possible.

Their key promoting factor is that you will lose weight, have more energy and just be happier. Don't fall for it! Starving your body back to health will cause acid to draw closer to vital organs and inevitably disease will manifest. This is a principal of truth that none of these industries will inform you of!

What is more is that, once again, it has that element of "diet" where you psychologically think and associate deprivation which sets you up to self-sabotage. These industries have twisted the whole meaning of the word "diet" so that now it has become the exact formula to pre-calculate weight loss disaster.

D - Depriving

I - Individuals

E- Every

T- Time

Will you lose weight? Sure, but you will also be burning lean muscle in the process and as you know the heart too is a muscle that is so vital for human existence. You would not want to jeopardize weakening that muscle just to shed a few pounds that will come back anyway once you resume eating solid foods again.

What about the popular South Beach Diet created by cardiologist Dr. Arthur Agatston? That too is one diet that appears to be a little more superior compared to others at the moment. However, it does bring to mind a rather peculiar thought about how a cardiologist could be taken seriously as an authority on nutrition. We all have figured out by now that the vast majority of medical doctors are no more nutritionally literate than the average Eve or Steve. Through their years of medical school, they often do not receive any appropriate training on foods, nutrients, minerals and the benefits of such for the human body.

Across the US and other countries like, Canada, Europe and Australia, there it is not really a requirement that doctors learn nutrition before they become licensed and begin to practice medicine. Most medical schools do not teach nutrition lessons. Astounding is it not? There is a Galactic enterprise of information out there on nutrition as it relates to good health and, at best, doctors may receive a whopping 60 minutes of training on nutrition. Hippocrates puts it best when he stated over 2,300 years ago, "He who does not know food, how can he know disease?"

So is it really likely that a cardiologist would know what is best to address the pervasive obesity issue, while keeping people as healthy as possible through and through?

One can only draw their own conclusions on the matter with this South Beach diet as they peer into some of the many inconsistencies in the book that makes a spectacle out of such misunderstanding of proper nutrition.

One puzzling example is: In the book (in phase 2 of the diet plan), he includes bananas as foods to avoid. Yet one of the recommended desserts is sliced bananas dipped in sugar-free (likely toxic artificial sweeteners) chocolate sauce. The good doc later advised that whole intact foods are better for you, but then on the other side of the neck mentions that mashed potatoes are better than whole baked ones. Those facts can be found on page 54 of the book.

This kind of nonsense is the same rhetoric that every diet out there is serving up and people are gobbling it up like they are at Hometown Buffet smorgasbord all-you-can-eat. This applies to anyone and everyone that is desperate to lose weight by any means necessary, and/or who has been in the dark about the real deal.

Get it into your head, get it into your mind and into your soul for the love of God, that losing weight cannot be the main focus for permanent changes. Period!

Focus on recapturing and/or maintaining your health. Employ the correct method and the weight will disappear forever. Rehabilitate yourself from the "Dietitis Syndrome" that causes symptoms of regurgitating weight loss myths. You need to move forward and get to see the authentic YOU that is being held captive by obesity and sickness.

Weight Loss Surgeries: Gastric Bypass and Lapband

There is a new wave of desperation evolving in an attempt to shed unwanted fat. A gentleman in Arizona who has been trying to shed about 50 pounds unsuccessfully has decided that he is so desperate that he is going to switch gears and instead try and gain another 50 pounds. This is so that he can be a grand total of 100 lbs overweight and thus qualify for surgery. He just wants to be thin again. There was a time when Black folks would not go under the knife for vanity purposes or otherwise. However, that has all changed thanks to Star Jones and Al Roker who have broken the mold for us.

"To butcher or not to butcher?" – That is the question.

Out of frustration and prodding from our medical community, we are resorting to getting butchered to get the weight off. This surgery is the gastric bypass surgery and lapband surgery. No matter how you slice it - or in this case whom you slice, it is dangerous and disrespectful to manipulate the body parts that were custom designed to suit our human needs. Doctors are playing God. While there is a time and place for surgery, in some instances when is going *too* far more than a notion?

The gastric bypass surgery involves stapling off or re-routing a small pouch from the rest of the stomach and attaching it to the small intestine. This will decrease calorie absorption because only a small amount of food can fit in there. The stomach is reduced to the size of two tablespoons. Before considering this method as a solution to end all your fat person woes, consider this:

There are leakages at two different connections from the incisions that you will have to heal from.

You end up with nutritional deficiencies and digestion problems, which can lead to a variety of other health complications very quickly. This contributes to why many people who undergo this type of surgery tend to look haggard with their faces sunken because of losing structural fat. Lean muscle has gone away leaving them looking deformed and disfigured.

Since they have to re-route the bowel, it creates potential blockages down the road that you have to deal with FOR LIFE per Dr. Andrew Larson who happens to be quite skilled at performing these kinds of surgeries. One coach at Notre Dame University almost lost his life from undergoing bariatric surgery. Don't take that chance unnecessarily with yours.

According to Roland Sturm, Economist for Rand Corp. (a non-profit organization group), the use of bariatric surgery has made no noticeable dent in the trend of morbid obesity. This overzealousness of these doctors and the attitude of "when in doubt, rip it out", is what is being nationally propagated.

Since there has been so many reports on the dangers of bariatric surgery, lapband has been pushing it's propaganda that it is so much better and safer. The explanation is that unlike the bypass, lapband only restricts the opening to the stomach by strapping your stomach with a band that is much like a belt buckle. The band works by decreasing the amount of food the patient can eat at one time. They are even toting a few token Black folks to endorse this preferred method of butchery. When are we going to realize that when man starts tampering with things he ought not, we end up with a whole heap of extra problems? We tell our little children not to play with rubber bands around their wrist, but yet we are allowing them to put one on their stomachs right along with us. Just a thought!

There is a study in the Journal of Neurology that described 27 cases of women and 5 men who developed a complication of a condition associated with weight loss surgeries. This condition involved symptoms of frequent vomiting, effects on the brain/nervous system, double vision, eye movement abnormalities, walking and memory loss. The study found these symptoms to appear after all types of weight loss surgeries.

Another complication of these surgeries is blood clotting because of the combination of being obese and having to be bed-ridden after surgery. Blood clots form in the legs or in the lungs, which if it's the lungs it can be deadly. All weight loss surgeries change the body's biochemistry. Once the body's biochemistry has been altered, any number of illnesses can sprout up. Why even put ourselves out there for that risk? We have enough ways to die without even trying!

What a great way to address obesity and its related illnesses by sending the message that it is still okay for them to not learn how to eat properly, moderately and sensibly for good health. So go get this surgery, eat what you want, you don't get fat again but you still end up with a disease ridden body from unhealthy food choices - only a skinnier one!

We haven't even talked about the cost in terms of the almighty dollar. The cheaper of the two is the lapband starting from $12,000 to the upwards of $30,000, not including follow-up visits around $200 each visit. Mo' money, mo' money and mo' money. It is understandable why the president of The Obesity Society stated that he sees the future as combined therapy with surgery and medication and other approaches used simultaneously.

Surgeries along with all other types of weight loss protocols, procedures, plans and the like should be heavily weighed and considered for complications, side effects and overall effectiveness. It is your body, you have to live with it - or be without it! Whatever the case, just be informed.

Now we have a fuller spectrum of the problem of obesity with all these external factors that exacerbate the issue for us a community.

- We know more about the role that the government and food industry play.

- We know why diets don't work for us (and anybody else for that matter) due to their approach being all wrong.

- We know that obesity is due to an abnormal function of some part of the body being unbalanced, many times caused by the very foods we eat and their toxic chemical substances.

Diets categorically cause imbalances within the body, and we're not interested in a temporary fix for obesity.

The picture is becoming clearer and clearer that in efforts to solve this obesity crisis these band aid remedies only serve to correct that one problem while creating hundreds more. Despite this, the time is ripe for us to let go of these fads and myths and learn to embrace the truth – especially to the truth that we as a culture must look inward for.

This is where personal responsibility comes into play to bring this whole epidemic of obesity full circle. Once again when specifically looking into facts surrounding Blacks and obesity, we must address issues indicative to our community. Since we lead in incidents of obesity, certainly we must have some unique concerns. We will continue to make minimal headway in the treatment and prevention, if we don't recognize these issues instead of turning a deaf ear to such.

Psychology/Perceptions

For African Americans there tends to be certain factors that play a role in our food choices such as our history, religion, our culture, friends, family and our environment. Let's talk about three in particular.

1) **Culture.** Studies show that Blacks are more accepting of larger body sizes than any other race. For instance, the University of Maryland explored eating attitudes, behaviors, psychology and ethnic identity comparing Black and white female college students. They noted that the biggest factor for the lower incidence of restrictive

eating disorders was primarily due to cultural differences in definition of beauty. While on one hand this seems to be a good thing, it has ended up hurting us more because our tolerance of these larger body sizes has caused us to be more obese than ever and subsequently lead to more obesity/health related illnesses.

We may think that we look fine - as in a sister being labeled "PHAT", or a brother being pleasantly plump as a show of prosperity and how well his lady is taking care of him. The fact is that it's not a cute thing when we know what this is leading to. Still you have a whole generation of folks in denial, citing they are not fat, just "big boned". Let's squash this fallacy right now, there is no such thing as "big bones".

Typically, many black women who think like that have a deep seated attachment to their fat which is difficult to shake when they are intelligent and successful. When delving a little deeper, it is often found that there is an underlying fear that losing weight will cause other women to be jealous of them.

In addition to that, they feel that men will tend to be more attractive to their figures instead of their character. We don't need to call folks out, but there are several high profile African American women who fit into this category as they revere themselves as Big and Beautiful. In actuality, they are just flaunting their obesity.

Due to these various lines of reasoning, it has led to an overall tendency to feel less guilty of overeating, thus making it less likely for us to change our diet and exercise. Statistics show that while 78% of Black women are overweight and 72% of Latina women are overweight, white women are far more concerned about weight (Abrams, Allen, Gray 1993). Ironically in the same University of Maryland study that was conducted, it was found that both Black and white women alike experienced high rates of depression, anxiety and low self-esteem.

Last, but not least is the common myth in our culture that once you have a couple of babies that somehow you earn the right or a free pass to be overweight. Either this is okay for some, or at minimum it is acceptable to carry around that inter-tube in the middle area, chalking it up as "baby fat". So the concept is to just accept that if you have children, you're body will not ever be as nice as it was prior to.

This is so erroneous, but our "culture" has cultured up and passed around this general belief. Note to self: Just because you don't personally know any mothers who have had children and are in shape; it doesn't mean they don't exist, and it doesn't mean that you can't accomplish this.

2) **Environment.** Our environment influences, not only our choices in foods, but also our ideals on exercise and physical activity. As touched on earlier, in our neighborhoods we have these carryout stores and mini-markets that only offer us fried fatty foods laden with sodium. They are processed foods inundated with chemicals that give these foods their flavor, color, and sweetness. Just because this is what we are offered, it doesn't mean that we have to accept it. Even if we're low-income and receive money

from the government to buy food, we still get to choose what we buy and where we buy it from.

Don't frequent Joe's Carryout to get wings and fries, Chen's Chinese to get pork egg rolls, or Julio's Cocina for overstuffed burritos. Instead, go to the supermarket and carefully select healthier foods by taking the time to read labels to determine the nutritional value in foods. The government can not take that freedom of choice from us. We have control over that and simply have to assume the personal responsibility individually. If we don't have to depend on money from the government, than we have an even greater responsibility in terms of making healthier food choices. We may be in the position to go a step further, and switch to purchasing from a local health food store.

What about our ideals regarding exercise and physical activity within our outside environment? Maybe we shy away from walking because of being in the 'hood'. Well, here are some extremely practical suggestions:

✓ We could choose to do group walks during the day.

✓ Put extra effort in household chores to increase physical activity.

✓ Play and horse around with the kids.

✓ Cut the grass, and maintain your garden.

✓ Dance to music in the house or at your favorite club.

✓ Go skating or bicycling regularly and consistently.

✓   Go swimming as weather permits, or do so indoors.

Just keep it moving, and the more you do - the easier it gets and the more it becomes a part of your life's daily routine. Choosing two or three of these activities for 30 minutes respectively each day will get you some amazing and lasting results.

3) **Family.** Lastly, the most important culprits are our family and upbringing. What we're taught as children from our families sets the tone for our food choices. For us as a community, our family tradition is the eating of "soul food". Food in general has always been the center of family interactions in the African American culture, particularly on Sundays. Studies show that 60% of us love to cook and spend an average of 47 minutes just in the preparations of extravagant meals. This is compared to only 29% for other races.

Nothing is wrong with this tradition in and of itself, but there is a problem with the less active lifestyle in combination with the fact that this soul food diet is laden with high-fat content, sugar and sodium for flavor. Continuous consumption of these foods without adequate exercise, and no regard to portion sizes, presents an added challenge to overcoming weight gain. We will revisit the proper way to exercise in an upcoming chapter and introduce a fresh new approach that is sure to help all of us whatever stage we're at with our level of physical fitness

Many of our families are at a lost for how to make nutrition a top priority, and this gets passed down generation to generation. This is why obesity in our youth is officially out of control - not just in our community, but other races as well. However, again, Blacks lead in the highest percentages of obesity cases in children; in fact all age groups. These facts we have been looking into are those indicative of our people.

Have you ever heard of the phrase "stinking thinking"? This is a mindset and way of thinking that is counterproductive, negative in connotation and paralyzing. It's called "stinking thinking" because it's a line of thinking that is foul in nature that doesn't belong in our heads. Instead, it should be thrown away and burned forever. What does it sound like? It sounds like, this, "Uh, uh, this is way too much money to be spending (on a health program)". The right line of thinking should be that a good health program is nothing more than paying "health assurance".

"I just cannot afford to go the natural route, so I'll just go with the meds," many say.

Wake up brothers and sisters! When are we ever going to get to the point when $100 or $200 is not a lot of money at all to spend on our most precious asset (our health)? For we are so very worth every penny.

If we don't pay now, you can bet on all the money some of us have lost in Vegas that we will indeed pay later!

Or when books or articles come out to give you suggestions on health-related matters or self improvement – we say, "Oh they are just trying to sell something." Then some will take there stinking thinking a step further and try to dissuade others from getting healthier by saying things like, "Oh so now you think you better than us?"

These statements are made by a lot of people - All because someone no longer choose to be fat, sick and hold onto a poverty mindset which makes one think that they can't afford to get themselves well.

When you choose to have a mindset of lack and scarcity, that is what you shall have - lack.

If the stinking thinking has been apart of your life, it's time to take out the trash. You have had your face in the poop, and maybe have been in it knee-deep. So, you know it stinks, but now you can move on past it. It is time to encourage one another even if we don't fully agree or understand them. If you don't like it - fine. Let that be for you, but don't knock what other people are brave enough to explore.

We either INFECT people or we AFFECT people. You make the call!

The sum total of the matter is this: We definitely have some noteworthy challenges. However, it's nothing that we cannot overcome. We only need to be completely aware of all the different dynamics that play into the weight loss cycle. We should be absolutely clear on the fact that obesity is a disorder that is a result from imbalances in some part of the body that needs your undivided attention and focus to correct.

We need not buy into misconceptions that obesity is only caused by overeating and lack of exercise or a curse from our relatives in the form of genetics. While we duly note this is true in some cases, we've come to realize the full picture encompassing other factors such as: social, environmental, and the government elements that should be assessed and addressed appropriately.

Another major element is the emotional/mental factor. A lot of us tend to eat out of nervousness, boredom, stress, and/or depression. The psyche of our people has indeed been warped by our own jaded perceptions of our overall health and well being. We must be informed on the mental and emotional repercussions of unhealthy eating and living. Let us again delve a little deeper into the real reasons of such emotional and mental instability of the ties that bind us.

Have you wondered to yourself why you may initially be excited about starting a new healthier way of living, only for the excitement to dissipate soon after? Or maybe you never even started due to lack of motivation? This was simply because you had unhealthy brain chemistry. Sickness and disease must be treated with a whole body approach which includes obesity.

Unhealthy brain chemistry leads to self-destructive behavior that is directly associated with bad food choices and lack of vital nutrients within the body and brain. What is even more important to note is that this process manifests itself differently in males and females. When men have nutritional deficiencies they are lacking in a chemical in the brain called dopamine.

Dopamine gives us energy and motivation. When dopamine levels are low in men, they will tend to seek out certain activities and engage in behavior that will stimulate the production of that chemical.

Then too, they won't do the things they should do for themselves due to lack of energy and motivation.

When a woman has nutritional deficiencies, usually she is lacking serotonin, which is a chemical that relaxes us and helps us to just - chill.

Without adequate serotonin levels, a woman will experience strong junk food cravings and depression. These very important brain chemicals are produced from specific amino acids contained in the proteins that we eat. Without the proper balance of these brain chemicals, we will not have the materials within our bodies to motivate us to change old unhealthy habits. It's like filling your gas tank up with sugar instead of gas and then expecting it to take you on a cross country road trip. You won't get very far; if you get anywhere at all!

You see no one ever gets to the roots of the emotional/ mental aspects pertaining to *why* we do what we do, or *why* we don't do what we are supposed to. These explanations absolutely determine behavior skill patterns. The ultimate goal is for people to come to an accurate knowledge of such.

These imbalances of brain chemicals may be present in obese and thin men and women. It even could be true for some that are just trying to overcome some other health challenge(s).

Junk foods will give us quick energy and comfort, but the problem is that the results are short-lived. Not long after consumption, the production of brain chemicals lessens and then you hunger for more junk food again and again. The body knows that it needs glucose for energy and signals the brain to get it by any means necessary. Whenever junk foods are chosen, the blood sugar is spiked and thrown completely out of balance. This will always be the case when we consume foods that lack properly balanced nutrition.

On the contrary, if you can give your body and brain all required nutrients, blood sugar levels will stay balanced on its own. We must NOT ignore this intricate balance of brain chemicals in trying to get healthier and lose weight. This is also the reason why the weight loss rate for men differs from that of women. They could be on the same program, but will lose weight at different speeds and/or give up for different reasons.

Go figure: The food companies exploit us with their commercials saying things like "They bet you can't eat just one," or "You have a fever for the flavor of a Pringle." This is hardly anything to be proud about, but they laugh about it all the way to the bank while we sit strung out as food addicts over their products.

We cannot stress this enough!!! When you get proper nutritional supplementation, you will feel so liberated to feel no urge to overeat. Since your cravings are non-existent, you have more focus, and stress levels drop. Stabilized mood and energy levels are so high, that you feel like you are floating. You have more recuperative sleep and of course the ultimate brownie point – WEIGHT RELEASE!

According to Dr. John Gray PhD, all overweight women are serotonin-deficient. Hence, he has proven in his work that with increased dopamine, the individual experiences ongoing, unlimited clarity, pleasure, energy and motivation. Furthermore with increased serotonin levels, others can experience calm, comfort and fulfillment.

This proper balance of good brain chemistry can be achieved by eating the right foods and satisfying all nutritional deficiencies. This insight is very crucial to understanding the psychological challenges of achieving optimal health as a people, as individuals - men and women respectively.

You can read all of the information you want in your diet and exercise books with all the little do's and don'ts. You can vow to exert the will power to change your ways, however if one refuses to address the brain chemistry balance, it won't last if it ever can begin at all.

The brain is the seat of motivation that drives us to make needed changes. We can not get to our final destination if we don't fuel it properly first. Get the right level of nutrients into your body, and feed the brain. It, in turn, will command your body to do the rest, and you will have all the energy and motivation you need to continue on.

Dr. John Gray explains in great detail this process of achieving optimal brain chemistry in a book *The Mars and Venus Diet and Exercise Solution.* In that same book, he reveals how he himself experienced healthy weight loss through proper nutritional supplementation. His work also has been extremely beneficial in improving relationships with men and women once they have come to an understanding of healthy brain chemistry.

Your body is a temple for your spirit and emotions to find balance in the physical plane, but it must be in a healthy state so that it may accomplish that balance.

Slavery Correlation

We have covered a number of issues involved in why weight loss has been a constant source of confusion, frustration, challenge, debate and utter wonderment. Yet it's time to tie everything into why this is particularly unique for the African American people and us only. Others will not fully understand us and or hear us, until we give due consideration to the psychology of our own people. We as African Americans *are* different from others. Granted, all of our internal organs are physiologically the same as humans; black, white, Asian, Hispanic, etc; which is why we are able to have globally-used textbooks of the anatomy.

Nonetheless as African Americans it is obvious that we are different. Like a special birth mark on a baby that has been born into a family, so too African Americans in relation to the world maintain a figurative birth mark. They have one very distinct characteristic in comparison to any other U.S. cultural, racial or ethnic group.

We carry a psychological backpack filled with baggage of slavery times, post-slavery and discrimination. According to The Hunter Miller Group's research analysis, this fact has had and continues to have a profound impact on how African Americans see themselves in EVERY aspect of their lives.

This insight gives a close-up shot in the mirror into our innermost thoughts - shadowing the force that drives us to behave the way that we do.

It explains why we tend to make certain choices regarding our health and/or don't make certain choices that we know will benefit us.

Obesity and sickness is the new form of slavery for us! There is no "white" man yielding and cracking his whip anymore, but we have carried the baggage from that and thus have unknowingly created our own self-imposed slavery.

The ties that bind us today are sickness, obesity, and let's not overlook poverty. Too many of us that want to heal ourselves and save our own lives, find ourselves not having the monetary resources to do so. Let this thought really touch your core. The former slavery has long ended. How long will we allow that to be our story?

Slavery is a part of our heritage as we all duly note. However, this 21st century slavery need not be our legacy. It is now time for authentic solutions and resolutions.

We don't have to be prisoners in our own bodies. Knowledge and power are the keys to unlock the shackles. As people of color, our bodies are majestically built; our men and women alike. We just have to have the confidence and determination within ourselves that we can individually *choose* to enlighten ourselves to a better, more holistic approach to weight loss.

Don't expect the governmental/political arena, food or diet industry to provide a solution in our best interest. Again, diets only serve to give you a temporary solution.

Don't be fooled or sidetracked. A whole body approach is by far the most superior way to getting true lasting results. Taking a holistic approach allows you to address the underlying causes of obesity, as there are a variety that we have covered such as, cultural, governmental, environmental, social, lifestyle factors, lack of physical activity and in almost every person - imbalances in some part of the body.

These imbalances can include:

✓ **Metabolic Dysfunction**

✓ **Impaired Thyroid Condition**

✓ **Imbalanced Insulin Production** – which inhibits normal bodily functions necessary to control excessive weight gain.

In order to achieve successful weight loss, all of these factors must be assessed and properly addressed. It is the duty of your physician, if he or she is highly-skilled to check and test for these imbalances appropriately. However, you must insist on this for yourself.

Points to permanently store in your memory banks are as follows:

- Successful weight loss can not now and never be achieved solely through the latest fad diet or weight loss supplement.

- It can not be sustained without proper exercise combined with superior nutrition.

- Even 'eating right' is not enough these days in order to achieve optimal health. You need a blueprint that will get you where you want to be using the quickest, shortest, safest route with NO HOLES in the sidewalks!

Let's raise the bar to even a higher standard for achieving permanent weight loss and vibrant health status. We don't want to dance around in the ring of life anymore; that is, taking the risk of getting knocked out. We don't want to take small jabs at trying to defeat obesity and sickness. Instead, we want a one-two punch that will knock it out cold to where it cannot get up and overtake our people as a whole ever again.

During the compilation of this book, there has been a very passionate organization comprised of individuals within our community blazing the trail to help free our people from the likes of this new form of slavery.

This organization is known as The Underground Railroad 2 Personal and Financial Freedom (www.undergroundrr2freedom.com), led by Dr. Karen E. Copeland O.D.

Dr. Copeland and others are spearheading this movement to recruit health-conscious African Americans which she refers to as "runaway slaves" to impact world health and free the black community from physical pain, but also from financial pain as well.

Dr Copeland says, "We equally need to be freed of financial pain too, as poverty like mindsets are at the crux of why we don't prioritize our health and instead opt for the cheap route."

The movement, of course, is modeled from the original concept led by Harriet Tubman in the 1800's.

These freedom riders no longer want to see the black community enslaved and in the bondage of an unhealthy body and excess weight. They are, in fact, leading thousands to the freedom land of good health and greater wealth.

This organization will stop at nothing until the destructive genetic, social unhealthy mindset that has become a part of our evolutionary conditioning is forever eliminated!

The organization has its movement underway within the community to show others how to change the view that we have of ourselves and where we see ourselves fitting into the world structure.

If you are reading this book, you must ask yourself this question: Will you allow yourself to continue to be held captive?

Or will you indeed join the ranks of becoming a "runaway slave", refusing to accept obesity, sickness and poverty as a way of life or as your legacy?

You have the power. The time is *NOW* to end your own slavery to obesity. Relieve yourself from this blanket of oppression and begin to take charge of your life in order to feel better, look better, and be better than ever!

II.

DISCUSSION OF CHRONIC DISEASES AND ENVIRONMENTAL FACTORS

There is a toxic and overweight culture existing in this 21st century which has caused widespread chronic disease. The truth is: Back in the 1960's, a lot of these diseases didn't even exist. For example, acid reflux disease, Multiple Sclerosis - and the list goes on. Many of us have family members who have multiple disorders - like the color of the rainbow.

This discussion though, of chronic diseases is not an overview of all the leading diseases. You can use reference books for that. Instead, this discussion highlight ones that are overwhelmingly afflicting the black community and that are easily controlled through proper nutrition and exercise. We want to increase awareness that most of the time the prescription drugs that are given to us as a solution is actually part of the problem.

For instance, aspirin is encouraged by medical doctors to be taken for the prevention of heart disease. However, it is estimated that a regular intake of aspirin is responsible for at least 2,000 deaths annually due to stomach bleeding.

Not only does experience teach us that they create additional health problems, but for some ailments, non-prescription drugs and prescription drugs can cause what we all want to control - excessive weight gain. According to the International Journal of Obesity, obesity triggers include high blood pressure drugs, anti-psychotics, protease inhibitors to treat HIV, diabetes medications including insulin, and over-the-counter antihistamines. All of these have been linked to weight gain. Many more drugs increase appetite and slow metabolism, such as anti-depressants, oral contraceptives and estrogen replacement drugs.

Let's get right down to business to find out about all of these various implications. First though, we would like for you to perform a simple request for the sake of this discussion and its grave nature:

If you happen to be near someone else at the moment, look at them and tell them you love them, even if you don't know them. You might think that is a silly request, but in actuality it may very well wake them up to the reality that someone else on this planet cares enough about them, even if they don't care enough about themselves.

Consider the following statistics that tells our story and lets us know that we are in trouble. Before you read this though, understand that this book was specifically targeted and written for the benefit of the African American people in an attempt to explain why we have not been successful in losing weight; thus incapable of dealing with its related illnesses as a whole. The facts are the facts!

The majority of whites (57%) and Blacks (54%) are not even aware that Blacks suffer a worst health status as reflected by a lower life expectancy. Did you get that? Neither Blacks themselves, nor our white counterparts are even aware. This should not be, after all the information being put out there. That is why we have chosen to turn our attention to our community – first!

If you have ever flown on an airplane with a small child while they are going over their mundane safety instructions, they always stress that the adult puts their own safety mask on first and then put the child's mask on.

The reasoning is that you can be of no use to the child if you can't breathe and are dying. Thus, you don't save anybody, NOT yourself nor the child.

News flash: We are having serious trouble breathing and if we don't focus on putting our masks on first, we won't be around to contribute any good to the rest of the world. Make no mistake about it! We are needed, each and every one of us, even the unborn.

Take a look at what is restricting our breathing:

Heart Disease

According to Reuters and the CDC, researchers say that African American men are 26% more likely than white men to die from heart disease at a rate of 841 deaths per 10,000.

Heart disease has been coined the "silent killer" or even referred to as the "big one coming on".

Would you care to know the reasons that they cite for this anomaly? You guessed it. Obesity and lack of exercise was at the top of the list, along with limited access to health care and lack of quality food available in many areas. Other factors include job stress and depression.

Too often the medical establishment will put over-emphasis on cholesterol levels with heart disease, instead of getting to the root of the problem. Consider that cholesterol-lowering drugs will destroy your hormone and nervous system!

It as a well-known overlooked fact that vulnerable plaque is the primary cause of 85% of all heart attacks and strokes. Yet, conventional methods of detection such as angiograms are not even able to detect vulnerable plaque.

With regard to heart disease, why don't we all have a private moment of silence for all of our inspirational Black leaders who succumbed to this disease?

When he died, the late Gerald Levert, (who was overweight) had a fatal combination of prescription drugs in his system. This is one of the reasons why we need to change today, as we cannot afford to wait. We need to do this for each other, to get the weight off, and get healthy. We do not want to keep putting things into our bodies that are going to create more problems on top of our weight issues.

Alternative treatments administered by natural health practitioners include:

- **MRI (Magnetic Resonance Imaging)** - for detection of vulnerable plaque

- **Dark Field Microscopy** - which is a live blood sample viewed through a special microscope for a closer detection of blood clotting

- **Detoxification Therapy** – which rids the body of harmful substances that build up in the body and bloodstream

- **Chelation Therapy** - helps break up the vulnerable plaque. Said to be 93% more effective as a treatment for heart disease than conventional treatments.

Stroke

This health disparity is greater among African Americans than any other race, with a risk of twice than that of whites. Blacks between ages 34-54 are at four times the risk. More than 100,000 African Americans have a stroke each year. In fact, every 45 seconds on average, someone has a stroke.

An astounding 30% of patients that have a stroke have another stroke within 30 days of their first one, and 1/3 of them have recurrent strokes within two years of their first one. 38% of all women who have a stroke will die within a year. This is so shuddering and terrifying that it makes you feel suffocated just by the mere thought. You want to throw in a hug or two for the person that may be near you? The most common causes for stroke are high blood pressure and hypertension.

Alternative treatments for stroke are:

- Hyperbaric Oxygen Therapy (HBOT)

- Chelation Therapy

- Prolotherapy

Diabetes

Approximately 2.3 million African Americans have diabetes, out of which 1/3 is not even aware. This means that for every six whites, ten African Americans have diabetes. It is most common for middle age adults and black women to develop heart disease. They are twice as likely to develop blindness, and 2.6 – 5.6 times more likely to develop kidney disease according to the CDC. This kind of "shuga" ain't so sweet; rather it has the opposite effect of wormwood that leaves a bitter taste in all of our mouths.

Are the available prescription drugs improving matters? Consider this fact about diabetes drugs: They will destroy your liver and can give you a stroke or a heart attack!

One golden nugget of truth is that there is a life-saving mineral that your doctor hasn't told you about - Chromium. Chromium is *crucial* and *essential* for glucose control. When insulin levels go up, receptor activity goes down. Chromium helps to revive receptor activity thus maintaining glucose control effectively without adverse side effects. It also is extremely helpful in burning fat in increasing muscle mass, as well as managing cholesterol levels.

Alternatives to dangerous medications are listed below:

- **Chinese herbs** - astragalus, rehmannia and wild yam.

- **Hydrogen Peroxide Therapy** - administered to those who had never been treated with insulin or other drugs.

- **Detoxification Therapy** – administered by a licensed alternative health practitioner

- **Exercise** - necessary and extremely beneficial for diabetics since it simulates the proper function of insulin to open the muscles for glucose to enter. While doing so, break a sweat because this will assist weight control, stabilization of blood levels and oxygenation of tissues.

High Blood Pressure

African Americans experience HBP more often than whites with an earlier onset and to a more severe degree. Death occurrences in Blacks due to HBP are the highest in the world. Another thing that should alarm you is that there is a mineral deficiency with high blood pressure patients, but many doctors do not implement this in their practice. The harsh reality is that your doctor hasn't even planned to tell you about that mineral deficiency. Instead, they have chosen to prescribe medication that actually exacerbates high blood pressure.

Major health/food tips:

1) Immediately eliminate refined salt, (which is sodium chloride) from your diet - completely. Glass and sand has been found to be present in refined salt.

2) Switch to sea salt instead, as it doesn't have the same effects on the body as the latter.

Lupus

This is a disease that should in fact be called the "woman of color disease". Lupus is three times more common in Black women than in white women. You may liken it to being "self allergic", where the body attacks its own cells and tissues causing inflammation, pain and organ damage. Contrary to popular belief, this is easy to address as it is largely caused by nutritional deficiencies with a 100% correlation to food allergies. Thus, in Lupus patients they will have poor communication between normal cells and immune cells.

Biofeedback training has been helpful as treatment along with detoxification therapy, chelation therapy and the use of naturopathic medicine. Some good herbs to take are Swedish bitters and nettle.

It has been proven that people receive remarkable benefits with the modifications in their diet of these items listed below:

1) Fresh raw veggies

2) A good source of clean, quality protein

3) Live system enzymes

4) Live digestive enzymes

5) Omegas 3,6,and 9

6) Soil-based organisms

7) Dark green leafy vegetables

ADHD (Or ADD)

Common sense can show us how obesity can directly be caused by consumption of unhealthy, fattening foods our children are eating, but what about other health implications? Let us take a look at the childhood epidemic of ADHD (Attention Deficit Hyperactivity Disorder). Currently, 26% of all African American children are diagnosed with ADHD, according to the Journal of the Medical Association.

Based on the most recent studies, it has been revealed that 80% of children with ADHD are symptom-free within 2 weeks just by eliminating the very foods we have been talking about from their diets. Through the elimination of all white flours, refined sugars, and then replacing them with good nutrition – these children can be relieved.

Without getting into every little food bandit responsible for the degradation of good health, one proven cause for ADHD has been hydrogenated oils. They literally poison the brain and nervous system, and create birth defects. Hydrogenated oils block absorption of essential fatty acids and deplete nutrients, minerals and vitamins absolutely crucial for good brain health.

Based on this fact alone, the so-called disease, ADHD or ADD, is nothing more than labeling diagnoses of a pattern of symptoms that are clearly created by poor food choices.

What's hot off the press about this matter is: The Lancet study in 2007 was published online by the British Medical Journal. This study conclusively and scientifically confirmed the link between food additives and ADD. It proved that the children's diets that consisted of food additives were significantly more hyperactive with shorter attention spans than those not given those additives. In those cases, you could see a marked difference in the children's behavior within an hour.

On the contrary, according to another study conducted by Harris Interactive for McNeil Consumer and Specialty Pharmaceuticals, 61% of children's caretakers cited that the meds had helped to improve the children's symptoms.

The fact about that is 80% of children on meds for ADHD will still need it as teens and 50% will still need meds as adults. What a dreadful thought! Then it gets even better with the notion of having to deal with countless harmful, and in many cases, life-threatening side effects.

This is all, in the name of "treatment", for something that can easily be reversed without the use of drugs.

According to Dr. Fred A. Baughman - a pediatric neurologist – ADHD, depression, and others are fictional chemical imbalances that are being treated with drugs for something that does not exist. He feels that these drugs are poisonous and damaging every time they are administered. The side effect rate is 100%.

Furthermore, he asserts that this epidemic is a part of a greater scheme to fraud parents into medicating their children who are otherwise healthy and normal. The obvious question would be: Why would this be a part of any scheme?

You can certainly find out why by visiting Dr. Baughman's website at www.adhdfraud.org. However, the real question should be: Would you rather your child be symptom-free, with no side effects whatsoever or on meds with a range of side effects pretty much indefinitely?

Cancer

African Americans have the highest incidence of death rates overall for certain types of cancers such as colon/rectal/lung and bronchus cancer; particularly in African American females. Black men have the highest incidence of prostate cancer according to SEER (Surveillance Epidemiology and End Results). What is so frustrating is that you will have people arguing about why this book had to exclude other races and chose to target African Americans. Here are some of the very reasons, based on the latest statistics. This is not all coincidental. 35% more blacks die from cancer each year, as compared to the general population. The sheer masses of the numbers in relations to these disproportionate health disparities indeed tell a story of their own!

Obesity has a direct link to cancer incidence. Doctors concede that fat can cause cancer by holding onto chemicals and carcinogens (cancer-causing agents) along with cancer-causing food habits. One American Cancer Society study shows that up to 90,000 cancer deaths annually can be attributed to obesity and being overweight. Researchers speculate that increased production of insulin and estrogen stimulate the growth of cancer.

However, contrary to public opinion, alternative treatments do work and are readily available for this disease, and include: enzymes, herbs, and phyto-nutrients as combined therapy. In many cases, not only have they been more effective than drugs, but are also inexpensive remedies.

Here is a little secret that shows just how powerful nature is vs. medicine:

A Cornell University study indicated that phyto-chemicals in the skin of an apple inhibit production of colon cancer cells by 43%. To further bolster the validity of those findings, the National Cancer Institute reports that foods containing flavenoids like an apple can reduce the risk of colon cancer by 50%. (Journal of the NCI)

The problem with conventional methods for treating our people with cancer is that the half-stepping approach is being taken. This is the main reason why they are no more successful with the life expectancy once a diagnosis has been made, nor is the quality of lives enhanced after undergoing chemotherapy or radiation. While white women tend to get breast cancer at higher rates than black women, black women tend to die more often and don't survive as long even with traditional therapies. You can not combat cancer with the very thing that causes cancer. Does that make ANY sense at all?

Chemotherapy creates an illusory effect of progression by shrinking the tumor, but it does not kill "cancer stemming cells" that will only grow back. Instead, it literally destroys tissues in the brain, heart, and kidneys - causing permanent damage.

Also just as icing is put on a cake, the cancer drugs further create a toxic internal environment in our bodies that ultimately bombards and weakens our internal organs.

By now you should have determined that chemo and drugs happen to be the only way that conventional doctors know how to handle cancer - or maybe, want to handle it.

These methods only will provide a measure of relief for some, but more is needed. All naturopathic doctors agree across the board that a complete and thorough treatment of cancer should be multi-faceted in offering prevention, healing, as well as health advancement.

Destroying healthy cells is not health advancing in any way. Nor is it "healing" because without healthy cells the body cannot repair and heal itself. With even more drugs being administered in order to "treat" cancer, this introduces a whole host of other illness and needless suffering.

At the end of the day, drugs don't prevent anything except proper immune function. If they were so great, where are all the healthy drug patients?

Good news is this: Because you have taken the time to investigate and let your mind explore; even if momentarily, you are sure to find more effective, non-invasive methods used for treating cancer that is preventative, healing and health-advancing.

This must be made abundantly clear and put as blunt as possible. DON'T WAIT until you have been brought to your knees, tappin' and rappin' on death's door, before you decide you want to employ an alternative method of cancer treatment.

More specifically, you need to make a choice on which method you will go with from the "get go". You can't try the conventional method of chemotherapy for a few months and only after you're weaker and more broke up than before, then decide to walk into the naturopathic doctor's office and say, "I have cancer, I have already tried everything else and I'm ready to be healed!"

The whole point of why alternative medicine works is that it will allow your body to support its *own* healing process, but if it's too weak and deteriorating you are not giving it much to work with. A more natural approach that a naturopathic physician will have patients undergo for healing could include:

- Massive Cellular cleansing

- Raw foods

- Enzymatic Superfoods

- Powerful and potent Juicing programs

Like you would avoid the Bubonic Plague, similarly there are certain things that must be avoided in order to heal thoroughly. These include: staying away from all carcinogens (cancer-causing agents in foods), such as sodium nitrates (found in meats). Also, avoiding parabens found in personal care products like lotions, bath, sunscreen, deodorants, etc.

One must make a 180 degree turn with their diet and incorporate potent nutritional programs. This may sound daunting to some, but actually there are some great food programs that simplify this overhaul, while making it tasty and enjoyable.

Interestingly enough, our country's very own former President Ronald Reagan had colon cancer that was reportedly treated by Dr. Steven Rosenberg without drugs and surgery; instead a natural method was used.

Infant Mortality

This is the first leading cause of deaths in the black population, even before heart disease.

The early death rates for African American babies were a minimum of 2.5 times greater than that of other babies in every state. According to Kathryn Hall Trujillo, founder of The Birthing Project, "The fact that the U.S. buried more babies than soldiers during the last century is totally not acceptable and this inability to save our babies has to stop…now!"

What role do we as parents and mothers play into giving our babies a fighting chance to combat this uncertain world of sickness and early demise?

For generations, we have heard about the many benefits of breastfeeding our young versus formula feeding. This was not only for the obvious strong bonding between mother and child, but more importantly - for the various health benefits as well.

However despite all the advocating of breastfeeding done over the years, a government report shows an alarming low percentage of black breastfeeding moms. Dr. Yvonne Bronner states that the culture of breastfeeding has been lost. According to Surgeon General David Satcher, only 29% of all mothers breastfeed their babies. In addition, only 19% of black mothers breastfeed for a six month period, this is the most crucial time to do so.

Why should any of this matter to us? The reason is because breast milk is unequivocally the purest and most perfect food for the baby. This discussion has gone in depth about the effects of certain types of foods and how they affect our overall health. Obviously, food would be equally as important, if not more in warding off infection and early death for these tiny beings.

Countless studies and research has shown for years and continues to show that breastfed babies suffer fewer illnesses such as diarrhea, earaches, infections and even more serious illnesses such as diabetes, asthma, pneumonia, and childhood cancers like leukemia lymphoma.

The National Center for Chronic Disease Prevention and Health Promotion states that increasing rates of breastfeeding is a crucial strategy for improving children's health and promotes such in the CDC Guide to Breastfeeding Intervention. With the childhood obesity epidemic, research has now pointed to the fact that breastfed babies are shown to have a lesser chance at becoming fat later in childhood. Also, notable is the fact that breastfed babies' brains develop much faster than formula fed babies. This fact remains irrefutable.

It is well-documented that in the U.S. alone, respiratory infections in formula fed babies are triple the rate than that of breast fed babies. Equally staggering is that most of these types of infections along with others, represent 16% of U.S. infant mortality totals. A joint study between the U.S. and Canada revealed a doubled risk for childhood cancer of 1.45 - 4 times in those of formula fed babies who had not received breast milk for more than one year.

So what is the message here? The message is that while formula feeding serves its purpose as medically necessary for babies who are unable to breastfeed. Breastfeeding should not be taken lightly with regards to its life-saving value.

Do not allow any establishments to make you second guess the value of breastfeeding by telling you that formula milk from cows is better than breast milk. It's totally false as there are more than 400 nutrients in breast milk that are not found in formula. This being the case, formula feeding can not hold a candle to fully meeting the nutritional and immunity needs of babies in the manner that breast feeding does. When babies are not breastfed, this leaves them all the more vulnerable to many serious illnesses that are claiming their young lives.

If they do survive than it has a direct impact on the overall quality of health later on life. So mothers: We have the power to provide a very strong and vital support structure for our children's health and well-being that we do well not to sleep on.

We need to lay a good foundation of optimal health before conception even by taking care of ourselves. This will maximize the chances of survival for our young who are totally dependant on us to make right decisions for them to make it in life. Tomorrow will present its own set of obstacles and challenges to overcome. However, we can absolutely do our part in preserving this miracle of creating life and adequately sustaining it?

We were entrusted with this role for a reason and only a season, so let us consider all the ways we can make a difference in our children's lives and for future generations to come. For those that are unable to breast feed their babies for medical reasons, they too can still do a great deal to help support their baby's nutritional and immunity needs.

Such ones just need to avail themselves to the ongoing, latest research available to find out what dangers exist. They also need to determine what they need to do to protect their children and learn exactly what their tiny body's need by way of nutrition. Thus, by making good nutrition an integral part of the family's infrastructure right from the very beginning, we are saving their lives and even their offspring's lives. If we expect to maintain and sustain life at every stage of development, we should all remember that nature is always the best choice!

Blacks and Pollution – Overlooked Disease Connection

In the UK, a study was conducted by the Environmental Pressure Group that measured the amount of chemical toxins found to be in the blood of its participants.

Chemical substances ranging from pesticides, fire retardants, and DDT (which has been associated with cancers and nervous and immune system disorders) were present. While light is being shed on the matter of pollutants in that area, pollution in the African American community is not being addressed appropriately.

We need to be aware of the increased risk within our community in respects to pollution, so as to lessen the damaging effects in our lives and our offspring. Jet rocket fuel has even been found to be present in women's breast milk. A New York study found that pregnant African and Dominican women were regularly exposed to pesticides in their community known as organophosphates. This small amount of exposure has proven to be more harmful than once thought as they have found that pesticide-exposed children may experience diminished stamina and coordination, impaired memory and reduced creativity.

According to the Washington-based Black Leadership Forum, 68% of Blacks live within 30 miles of a coal fired power plant as compared to 56% whites. 30 miles is the distance within where people experience maximum effects from smokestack emissions.

Nationwide, 71% of Blacks live in areas that do not meet federal air and pollution standards as compared to only 58% of whites. There seems to be no rush to make it compliant either. Stricter testing should be enforced to assist in the detection and prevention of these harmful substances. There is ongoing research that suggests that due to melanin in the skin of Blacks, we tend to harbor more toxins that we need to be aware of. It's still too early to conclude anything more about this suggestion.

Another key factor as to why Blacks are harmed more by pollution is that Blacks are more likely to work in asbestos, textile, coal and silica mining industries. This is where they are over exposed to occupational respiratory ailments and these hazardous materials that contribute to chronic lung diseases. This explains the higher death rate from asthma in Blacks, being as high as 38.7% per one million deaths as compared to 14.2% per one million deaths in whites.

People testing positive for contaminated blood is proof that it is time for the government to address this pollution issue aggressively. This shows us that after years of exposure to these external environmental toxins, they build up and take their toll on our bodies. Not only are we at risk for illness affecting the lungs and the heart, but also for inflammation of the brain as well.

It is absolutely vital that we get stricter laws on pollution in our areas to stop this ongoing contamination in everyday life for the sake of our health, our children, and future generations.

However, we should not wait until the government steps in.

Why? In spite of the governmental protective laws for pollution, Blacks or people of color still bear the health burden of toxic soil, polluted water, and air.

Alternative treatment and diagnostic precautions could include environmental medicine, which explores allergens, air, water, soil, mold, dust etc…to address pollution-related illnesses.

Aren't most of us aware of these staggering statistics? We don't live in a bubble; surely we have heard some talk of the effects of this toxic, polluted world. What we may not have known though for sure is that a lot of these "symptoms" of a much greater problem, are not guaranteed to be our future just because there was either a family history of such or because it's a part of our environment.

What should become increasingly clear at this point in the discussion is that there are some major disconnects here. We have disconnects in the governmental protective laws and the American medical system in understanding and, of course, admission to the link between diseases and nutrition. There are disconnects between disseminating the proper information to the African American people. We have already received an eye opener about the disconnect of the American health care system and how it has sorely failed to do its job for us all. This is seen in the documentary *Sicko*.

As for the African American sector, for years we have known that we have been given a raw deal when it comes to adequate health care. For us it has been down right deplorable and operates really more from a model of "sick care" instead of health care.

So many have given up going to the doctor because they feel that they wont be treated fairly anyway. Dr. David Blumenthal, director of Harvard's Interfaculty Program on Health Systems, stated in a report conducted by the Institute of Medicine that members of racial/ethnic minorities are given lower quality health care than whites even when they make as much money and carry the insurance. According to Target Market News, Blacks alone spend approximately 18 billion dollars in health care annually. We certainly are due better treatment than what is currently offered to us.

In 2003, according to Reuters the Washington Journal Health Affairs reported in a study that Blacks and Hispanics feel that they receive a lower level of care. Even 1 out of 5 whites felt that minorities get shortchanged. The poll's findings show that there is a persistent feeling among us that the care we are getting is not equal to that of whites. This is the way things still stand today. It is what it is, so in the meantime do we wait for things to change?

The information that somehow manages to be received has become nothing short of a colossal challenge to get the African American population to follow through on what is being advised. There are thousands upon thousands of books, tapes, seminars, health advocates speaking out on what we all should be doing for good health and the right foods we should be consuming. All of this is nothing more than recycled information. The same "you know what", warmed over!

Why do these numbers continue to rise despite all the "knowing all about it" going on? All the education on prevention, all the workshops for treatment, all the latest drugs and surgery options, revisions on various health care systems, why are we still not in better health? Today's society has the most doctors, hospitals, drugs and medical technology than ever before in history. Our compass is broken, we are lost and going in the wrong direction. Either as a race or as a whole, something is undoubtedly missing. So we need something that will help us get back – true north!

The answer is so simple, that it is sickening - literally! What's being done to supposedly solve these problems is NOT working.

Doing it their way, doing it your way, doing your own thing has gotten us in the trouble we are in now - SICK, SICKER, FAT, to MORBIDLY FAT and for others that cannot speak for themselves - DEAD.

Other ethnicities right here within this country have either already figured it out, or are well on their way to.

What about us? Why haven't we done so? Yes, we have gathered from this discussion that there has been a greater scheme of things at work and that this has been the case for most of our history. We are the last on the totem pole to get enlightened on such matters. Secondly, even though some of us may already know about the inner workings of the big money schemes that perpetuate bad food choices, when it comes time to translate into action – nobody does anything.

We still continue on eating those habitual foods that we have already talked about. For emphasis: high fatty, salty, processed foods, refined sugars and more.

To get you in the ballpark, there was a truck driver who decided that he wanted to make a lifestyle change because he was diagnosed with hypertension. He was to start out trying it for a 30-day period. Of course, he had weight issues that he wanted to overcome. He started eating healthier, more balanced meals, drinking more water and within about 4 weeks time was able to lose 22 pounds. Most importantly, when he went back to the doctor's office to check his levels, it was normal. Naturally he was quite happy about that. However after the 30 days was up, he decided that he no longer wanted to continue on with this lifestyle change. The reason being was that he did not want to give up his pork chops and other parts of his high-fat, salty diet.

Sadly, this is the typical scenario within our community and in the world in general. There is a definite reason for this too. For most of us, some unhealthy condition could initially motivate us to get started on a health program or regimen in an attempt to avoid the misery of some ailment. However, half way into the regimen, it's soon realized that in order to be symptom-free you have to continue to have that perfect diet; absolutely no dairy, no sugar, no bread, no processed food, or fat etc.....

These can be very restrictive and quite extreme. So once a person begins to feel better or lose the extra weight, they relax and go right back on a more tasty and delicious; but not as healthy diet. They conclude that it is way too burdensome to do something that perfect, so why even try? That no longer has to be the case.

Before the conclusion of this book, every African American living and breathing will have the opportunity to learn, not how to follow yet another "perfect" diet for healthy eating, but instead learn to live a completely healthy, balanced life. We will learn how to focus only on installing healthy eating habits as opposed to kicking bad ones. What you focus on expands and you get more of it. That is why we no longer want to focus on all the bad habits to get rid of, but shift the focus to the implementation of good habits, so we can get more of them.

This will help all to put an end to benign ignorance, and at that point no one can blame the government or anyone else for why they are overweight, sick or dying. You can blame one person: YOU. Once you have knowledge on any given issue, there also comes accountability and responsibility.

The single most effective secret to wellness for our time and all time will be revealed, and will empower every individual that chooses to trust his or her own God-given common sense to utilize it.

He (the creator) of all life implicitly tells us that he teaches us all to benefit ourselves. We were all given free will to decide for ourselves to make the best choices for our health and everything in between. It was never intended for it to be the sole responsibility of the doctor, who clearly has shown little or no regard for his handiwork. Instead, doctors think that they do a better job.

We can not and will not make the wisest decisions though if we are blinded, close-minded and/or brainwashed. This is the time for us to shake ourselves out of this mental myopia and cultural hypnosis we have been living in.

For far too long, we have been content with playing the victim role knowingly or unknowingly - believing that the only way to deal with obesity and sickness is through drugs and surgery. We have been conditioned by the medical establishment to believe that disease is caused by genetics, and/or that the only way to correct it is through conventional methods of treatment.

It has been already determined why this is so and that is because there are financial gains involved in every step of the game that outweigh any loss of lives that are incurred in this situation. They get to sell more drugs to "treat" disease indefinitely, without ever getting to it's true origin. Because of widespread obesity coupled with chronic disease, they get more bang for their buck by offering us a lifetime membership within the drug club. They can continue to generate even more money off more drugs, and in some cases for fictitious diseases. All the while, they are hijacking the personal power of the patients who think they will get and/or stay healthy from taking drugs. There is that blind trust again!

To illustrate this, note how the movie script plays out where Blacks star as the main characters. We feed ourselves junk - day after day, week after week, year after year - thus making the food companies richer. These foods as noted earlier are nutritionally inferior. The plot thickens when we continue to lead less active lifestyles. This will, in turn, provide the perfect breeding ground for obesity and related disease. We then run to the wide-open arms of the medical industry that has sworn under oath to make us feel better. The medical industry, by means of the pharmaceutical industry, will coax us into taking manufactured drugs to mask the symptoms of disease caused by food we bought and consumed.

So, then you get this wonderful jail sentence with an imprisonment term for life of taking drugs that only provide short-term benefits, with significant risk causing you to sacrifice long-term health. This completely violates the first rule in medicine: *First, do no harm!* All the while, the doctor fully supports the production of this movie by giving "Siskel and Ebert"- type rave reviews, telling you that this is okay. Then, the FDA gives the final round of applause by signing off on it.

The thing that has been so mind-blowing, is that the FDA is overly aggressive at making sure that healing herbs are banned while deadly drugs are totally legal and handed out like penny candy. This is a good rule of thumb! If you have a doctor that only wants to give you a prescription every time for everything, you should change your doctor. These doctors have graduated from the mentality of, "Take two of these and call me in the morning," to "Take 5 or 10 of these, and don't bother calling me until you have a different problem."

Let us clarify this though, as a side point that not all doctors are "pill-pushin" pimps who behave this way of being money hungry and careless. We know there are some out there who take their craft seriously, and really want to make a difference in the world. Because many lives have been saved due to such individuals, we would like to acknowledge them and encourage them to continue searching for better, new and improved methods to treating patients as safely as possible - one day preferably, without prescription drugs.

At the rate we are going now with so much suppression of information and/or lack there of, it is predicted that by the year 2012 - 1/3 of Americans will have diabetes. The pharmaceutical industry earns $1,300 per month per person from diabetes testing and medication. So that is millions of people times $1, 300 per month. That is way too much money just for one chronic illness. As for cancer, USA Today reports that publicly traded corporations have only one goal and that is to increase profits, which means selling more drugs.

According to the Associated Press, drug companies are seeing that cancer can be quite lucrative and plan to make billions of dollars in profits by selling cancer drugs.

Here are some other facts for you:

1) On average, doctors in this country receive $13,000 - $500,000 per year from drug companies.

2) The medical and pharmaceutical industries are allied partners in this big money business scheme. The FDA gets paid in a major way, collecting over $200 million dollars per drug approval.

3) There is an act called PDUFA (Prescription Drug User Fee Act) that has been in effect since 1992, which allows money to be paid to the FDA so they will review and approve drugs.

4) There is always a rush to approve new drugs without extensive testing for safety due to loss of revenue. This is the case because every day a drug is held up from marketing represents a loss of one to two million dollars in profit. Here is an interesting comment on the subject matter: "It's shocking, how can you say, release drugs to the market sooner, and not know if they're killing people... it really is a dramatic statement of public priority." Dr. Brian Strom MD, Chairman of Epidemiology University of Pennsylvania.

5) Since drugs are put out on the market to people despite threat to consumer safety, drugs that are FDA approved are estimated to cause 25,000 deaths outright every year in the U.S. alone and contribute to another 115,000 deaths each year.

6) Medical malpractices cause another 100,000 deaths annually.

We all have assumed that the FDA's job is supposed to protect us as consumers, but really all the facts seem to be telling us otherwise. It appears that they are working for the pharmaceutical industry instead, by way of protecting them. They have made it their business to protect drug company profits and of course their cut of the dough. ($200 million plus). That leaves us (the American people) out in the cold with no appropriate protective wear. We ultimately shiver to death from such neglect and greed.

The damages that drugs can do, will outweigh it's hoped for benefits!

The FDA's very own senior drug researcher David Graham testified before Congress that the FDA is incapable of protecting the American people.

He further asserted that tens of thousands of people are injured or killed because of the FDA's disregard for safety. Needless to say he is considered to be a shameful whistleblower for his publicly speaking out about such before Congress.

Consider some undeniable evidence to support these claims:

1) In 2004, the FDA was found guilty for suppressing a report written by drug safety in an advisory committee meeting that proved that most anti-depressants don't work for children.

2) FDA approved anti-depressant drugs can make you psychotic. They are mind-altering drugs that impair children's learning capabilities and increase risk of violent, aggressive behavior. Also, noteworthy in this regard the Columbine shooters were found to be on such meds.

3) The FDA actually lobbied against another country (Canada) to keep dangerous ADHD drugs on the market even after fatalities occurred.

4) The FDA approved the dangerous drug Vioxx and there was a jury verdict for $253 million against Merck for the damage and loss of lives.

5) Coumadin, a commonly prescribed drug used as a blood thinner, has been responsible for more deaths than any

single drug currently on the market, according to David Graham.

In September 2007, an article was published by Harvard Health Publications about a poll conducted by the Mellman Group and Public Opinion Strategies.

This poll found that 50% of Americans overall are skeptical and downright disturbed about the job the FDA is doing in protecting us all. In the same report, James Thurber PhD of the Center for Congressional and Professional Studies was quoted as saying, "The FDA needs to do a better job about being transparent and open about what they do, and their findings."

If these facts haven't convinced you that something is seriously wrong with these drug companies, health care systems and regulatory agencies, maybe this will: A paper written by a group of medical researchers entitled, *"Death By Medicine,"* compiled government health statistics and medical journals to give never-seen-before, definitive proof of medical blunders.

According to Life Extension Magazine, these researchers - which most are licensed medical doctors have found that the total number of deaths caused by conventional medicine is around 783, 936 per year. This staggering number reflects a dangerously flawed system that should not be given blind trust by us (African Americans) or any other American.

So what is the point that we should gleam from this? The point is that we have to open our eyes to the fact that none of these entities have our backs. If we don't take the time to get hip to this deception and begin to search for other alternatives that are safe, effective and reliable for our health crisis, we very easily could be the next victim of their death-dealing deeds!

The current methods and approaches to promoting good health have resulted in extreme futility. To demonstrate this futility, you can liken what is currently being done as someone asking you for a nice tall glass of water on a sweltering hot day. They may feel that it is an easy enough request to fulfill. When they pull out the glass and begin pouring the water, they realize it has no bottom in it. How long do you think it would take to fill up the glass with the life saving water? You are absolutely correct; they would NEVER be able to do so. This is what futility with our current approach to illness and obesity looks like; only on a much grander scale.

By now you should be gathering that drugs will never make you healthy, but they will continue to make those entities (pharmaceutical, medical, FDA) very, very wealthy! If the profits from drugs are not lucrative enough for them, they have decided to have their hand in the profits of vitamins. Some pharmaceutical companies launch vitamin companies and/or buy out existing ones to get even more dividends off of selling pure "crap". So essentially, they are double-dipping their hands in the cookie jar.

When we talk about "crap" vitamins, this includes what they are offering our kids and calling it healthy vitamin supplementation. There are dozens of kid vitamins out there, but the top selling and most popular vitamins on the market for kids are Flintstones™ and Scooby Doo™.

These types of children's vitamins are supposed to be healthy for our kids to consume and fill in the gaps when our food can't supply proper nutrition. Yet, among listed ingredients they contain the very harsh chemicals we mentioned earlier including: chemical dyes, yellow #6, blue #2, red #40, aspartame, MSG, hydrogenated soybean oil, phenylanine and more. Remember when you combine two or three of these chemicals, it could easily be harmful. There products should contain 100% of *all* the vitamins necessary to fulfill nutritional deficiencies. Instead, they contain no zinc, no manganese and only 40% vitamin A. Despite their huge nutritional voids; they *profess* to be the *best*!

Its "crap", point-blank! Ask yourself if a children's vitamin is so good for them, why does it clearly state on the bottle, "Keep out Of the Reach of Children"? It's a kid's vitamin.

As African Americans, we need to inform ourselves in such a way so that we can become partners in our health care instead of being passive recipients, blindly accepting whatever is dished out to us.

We have the right to access all relevant information needed to make our *own* private health decisions whereby we enjoy the freedom of exploring alternative healing methods.

Why highlight this information? Why is it relevant? In order to find out why a current system in place does not work, you must look at the holes and gaps in it that prevent it from being full-proof - if effective at all.

Our society can continue to go back and forth over scientific discoveries and breakthroughs all day long. However, we say that when scientific theories or evidence is tentative and not conclusive on a matter, each of us should not hesitate to call on our own common sense for guidance. We should also not allow embarrassment to interfere with our reasoning on the truth.

If you only knew the truth, do you think that you could handle it? Will you accept it as being such?

Based on an article published by *TruthPublishing.com*, one vital truth is that certain foods or food-based nutrients either stimulate or suppress your genetic code turning on or off biological processes that control degenerative diseases.

The article went on to explain that this means that degenerative diseases such as diabetes, cancer, and others are not all to blame on our genetics. Now, we understand that every one of us has genetic health strengths and weaknesses that are different. This makes Rodney more susceptible than Denise to a certain disease. However, that in and of itself does not seal our fate that we will get the disease for sure.

There are over 8,000 statistics with correlations between diet and disease that prove otherwise. This is heavy! Not only that – it should make you feel empowered to know diseases are a consequence of action or inaction that we ourselves have control over. No, disease does not just happen to us! Once you have grasped this concept, your duty is to become educated about and understand which foods create which effects. You can read more about this in a book called *The China Study* by T. Colin Campbell et al.

There are studies that are on record right now that have proven that nutrition affects multiple generations. This revolution of life science proves that DNA is *not* the sole source of inheritance. This was identified as the study of Epigenetics conducted by researchers at Children's Hospital of Oakland Research Institute with Dr. David Martin.

They were able to determine that a pregnant woman's diet and nutritional supplementation can and will influence future generations' health. So, now more than ever it is imperative that we reinforce and boost our nutritional intake of super foods.

Furthermore, this enlightenment means that genes don't automatically manifest disease (with the exception of some rare cases).

Next, we have control over our health destiny through nutritional supplementation and by ridding our bodies of chemical pollutants. That is what the science of Epigenetics proves without a doubt - that diet and chemical toxins are the controlling factors of genetic expression. Here is the added bonus of these findings:

For all intents and purposes, we can be confident that just because your mommy, daddy, aunties, and uncles, are all overweight, doesn't mean you are destined to be so too.

This study of genetics hasn't even fully permeated other countries. Therefore, as Blacks we need to know about it.

There are still some pockets of the world that obviously don't know about these findings. For instance, based on a recent survey, 31% of women in Europe stated that they would undergo a mastectomy, removing both breasts if they knew they had a family history of breast cancer.

They already made a decision to be chopped up in surgery and don't even have cancer yet. How absurd! Instead of exploring other options or solutions to keep from going to such an extreme route, they do the opposite. Why? There are thousands of licensed health practitioners, scientists, researchers and even some MD's worldwide that know and treat people everyday through the power of natural health without drugs and surgery.

One such doctor is Lorraine Day, MD. She practiced medicine for over 20 years using conventional methods. Then she was diagnosed with breast cancer. After she refused to be treated with the same conventional methods of treating cancer such as radiation and chemotherapy, her colleagues sent her home to die. For she already knew first hand what those treatments did to her patients and did not want to share their fate. She was absolutely determined to do so without drugs and surgery, although that was what she was always taught in medical school to do for everything.

After conducting her own research (yes, even a doctor, an MD conducted research to re-educate herself), she began to understand that the body can heal itself when given what it needs. Dr Lorraine Day remains cancer-free to this day without drugs. Of course, she did this before opting for chemo and radiation which would have only accelerated her deterioration and weakened her ability to heal naturally.

Remember this key point:

Everything man ever needs is available through nature.

Another example was of bio-physicist Dr. David Walker, PhD when he reversed his cancer through natural methods. According to an article by author, Teresa Tsallaky - he was sued. Reportedly, he was actually helping others heal themselves and reverse disease safely and naturally, but they took everything from him and he ended up moving to Mexico. Because he had seen the transformations over and over again, he was not going to allow the U.S. government to stop him from saving lives. Due to his training as a biophysicist, Walker learned that cancer cells have high toxin counts. Also, people with cancer have low blood oxygen levels which cause cells to mutate. With this knowledge, he clearly understood the simple logic of counteracting the actual disease process of cancer. In doing so, he has proven that if you can recharge these cells, the body will heal itself. This is pure common sense ladies and gentlemen! Just like a cut or an open wound will heal on its own, so too will the body. Dr. Walker's protocol includes the following recommendations:

- **Detoxification Therapies** - many extensive methods available.

- **Bio Resonance Therapy** - an actual machine that recharges cells that have mutated.

- **Phytonutrients & Glycoproteins** - out of the nine glycoproteins essential for cells to reproduce themselves; only one is made by the body and food must provide the rest.

There are hundreds upon hundreds of success stories right here in your own backyard and abroad. You don't have to live in fear of this disease and feel there is no hope unless you go the conventional route. Be encouraged, thoroughly informed of all possible options and aware of your body's own "infinite wisdom!"

Likely, you are at a point in your reading of this information where you are asking the following questions: What is it that is so natural and so much more superior to other methods to help me get healthy, lose weight, have energy, vigor and vim for life? What could it possibly be that I haven't tried already? Why can't I just continue to follow the same old advice that has been given for years - eat right, exercise etc.? Why can't the proposed new solution just be spelled out right now, get to the point already?

All the above questions can only be answered in one way. If you are in fact thinking those things or asking those questions to yourself, that is precisely why more significant progress with your overall health have not been made.

This is not another book that is going to spend 300 pages giving you Do's and Don'ts or giving you a bunch of hype as to why you should be on this plan or that one. This is not another book that is going to load you up with a bunch of fancy health recipes or give you just enough information to tickle your ears and wet your appetite, leaving you in want of even more answers.

Learning how to get healthy and stay healthy is not about speeding through like some kind of NASCAR race. Rather attaining to good health is more like a journey where you embrace each step, recognizing and identifying potential potholes that could trip you up and cause you to veer off the road. Your peripheral vision must be sharp and on point to achieve this. This is not a magical process, and it takes time!

Speaking of magic, there is an informative best selling book out that is promoting a magic weight loss cure of HCG (Human Chorionic Gonadotropin). HCG is a protein hormone that is naturally produced in a pregnant woman's body during pregnancy. Now it is being used along with an extremely low calorie diet, to help the body burn stored fat and assist in weight loss.

What readers should note is that HCG treatment is far from being magical. If this should be a serious consideration to solve your obesity issues, understand that patients must be monitored by a physician daily, they must be weighed daily, injected daily and also MUST follow the perfect diet to the letter.

This is a very time consuming process and should be heavily thought through before proceeding. If you are more than 15 pounds overweight than buckle down because just for the 15 pounds of weight loss, you must undergo treatment for no less than 26 days. You can lose no more than 34 pounds at a time and then you have to wait for 6 weeks for the next series of injections, as the body will build up immunity to the HCG treatment.

Furthermore, this procedure is not for everyone and it is hardly curative unless the patient fully cooperates with the physician to the letter with no deviations; otherwise it can annul the effects completely. To annul the effects, simply means that the weight is regained. On the other hand, if you have the time to follow the protocol and you meet the prerequisites; that may be a viable, safe, alternative for you. On that note, one final thought is that if you are looking for any kind of book that is going to promise you "21 days to a skinny you", "shrink yourself in two seconds," or "101 different ways to gain more energy and be happy", you may as well close this book right now and put it into your cellar to collect dust! That may have sounded a little facetious or even crazy, but that is exactly what people have been listening and buying into - craziness in it best form!

Remember that kind of impatience and desperation is what has gotten us HAD to begin with. Wanting that quick fix, "magic" this, "money back guarantee" that. Research has proven that African Americans have a high propensity for instant gratification - which we seek to transcend!

In contrast, this book was intended to appeal to people's sensibility, reasonability through 100% integrity. We all want trusted, reliable sources of information. That is what has been delivered to you. The power to put choice and freedom with respects to our health on the front burner of our minds, has been the main objective.

The intention has been set to enlighten our people to higher levels of consciousness and encourage a paradigm shift in our thinking so as to make sustained lifestyle changes that can be passed down to future generations.

That can only be accomplished when we are able to sift through all the garbage that has been fed to us - literally, mentally and physically. This happens only when we have pulled out the weeds that defile our rich soil. During the reading of this entire book, we have been pulling out the weeds.

That also entails us to look at the big picture, the whole picture of why we haven't made greater strides as a people with our health.

Promoters and advocates of holistic health are having tremendous success where conventional doctors have miserably failed. These health professionals are helping people heal from all kinds of sicknesses, and are assisting others to shed weight safely, quickly, and naturally. This is happening just as sure as you are reading the words on this page - right this very moment. It's being done without the use of drugs, surgery, diets and injections.

This is not common knowledge, only because our voices in the holistic world are not being heard loudly due to the news media, and the propaganda from the government trying to suppress our voices.

Many don't want our voices to be heard because of fear of the truth to ring clearly, for all to hear. The million dollar question is, *why?* Our collective voice needs to and should be heard. There, is in fact, a revolution underway worldwide that we as African Americans have every right to be apart of - if we so choose. Yes, we can choose to be a formidable force to be reckoned with and make our presence felt.

Over to the left, you have the old institution of things or the (medical establishment) whose mind set is: one-size-fits all medicinal approach to disease - supported by billion dollar pharmaceutical companies, pumping out venomous prescription drugs back to back. They are shoulder to shoulder with the FDA, who sits back and collects the bank roll. All of them scratch each other's back by the act of masking symptoms vs. getting to the root causes of all illnesses - be it minor or serious.

The rest of the world knows, and now we have come to know that osmosis doesn't cause us to just wake up one day with diabetes or cancer. Rather, we give ourselves disease day-by-day from the way we eat, live and the way we manage stress.

Those on the right side - know this emphatically!

Over to the right, there is the new institution (or holistic establishment) who are enlightened warriors that possess the will and courage to question authority; recognizing that there is always more than one way of skinning the cat – treating disease. Even more importantly, they possess the realization that current methods aren't always correct. It isn't about bucking the system or rebelling against it, but just merely exercising one's own God-appointed rights as humans - free will. These individuals are not guided by popular public opinion, but instead pure objectivity as wise and discerning individuals. Yes, they are independent thinkers! These are the people who believe in healing by natural means and who know synthetic, laboratory made drugs are toxic and cannot do the job better than natural agents.

This growing sector of individuals knows that in many, many cases diet and lifestyle alone can be the best cure.

What do we do to get on board and not miss the boat?

How do we begin to affect a change in ourselves - first?

So for starters, you must UN-learn destructive behavior. That is the first step to recapturing your health or anything else we truly want in life that has remained elusive to us.

There are two main steps in the corrective thought process towards un-learning destructive, disease-causing behavior patterns.

Step 1- Awareness

Fortunately throughout this entire book, we have been growing your awareness. Therefore, you have a head start in the first step in this process, simply by reading this book. The first step to all change is, in fact, awareness. If there is one single thing that can take you out of the game before you even begin is thinking that you have it all figured out.

Having a three-word-phrase in your everyday vocabulary can cause your journey to wellness to come to a grinding halt: I-already-know. Know this - that if you continue with that line of thinking and continue to do what you always have; your physical health and well-being will slowly begin to deteriorate. You will get more sickness and disease on top of obesity and will watch your energy levels continue to plummet before your very eyes.

If you are a health professional with your fancy titles and all your "degrees", yet *think* you already have the answer to treating illness, when was the last time you CURED and or eradicated disease from any of your patients? When was the last time you made them feel all better without the use of a manufactured drug that ended up giving them a host of side effects? When was the last time you helped a morbidly-obese person lose weight without cutting them open like a slaughtered pig?

When do you think will be a good time to get over all the medical school dogma and begin to think for yourself?

We are moving in a time where medical doctors can choose to operate from a different, more effective model of care where he/she believes illness is almost always caused by multiple factors and make every effort to treat the "whole" person. In doing so, they also believe it is best to treat the patient before symptoms appear. As an added benefit, it minimizes inflation of health costs. This approach is the real "preventative medicine"!

If your commitment lies in practicing your art with integrity and courage, and you are open-minded to the newest advances in the healing arts, despite it not being taught to you in medical school, it's possible for you to be counted amongst the network of doctors and health professionals that are in the forefront of this revolution. These leaders of the pack will guide others to freedom of health care. It is strongly recommended for those that have realized by now that they don't know everything, to read up on this in a book called *The Assault on Medical Freedom* by P. Joseph Lisa.

If you are just someone that happened to have tried all kinds of programs to lose weight, are you still over your desired weight goal? Has the weight come back?

Are you someone that has been on several medications to treat one persistent condition but you still have it, and are living with even more discomfort?

Did the doctor tell you that you will be fine just as long as you stay on the meds for the rest of your life?

The thing is, life was not meant to be lived in that manner and your own responses will tell you where your level of awareness is and lets you know that there must be something you DON'T KNOW. If only you would open your mind to other possibilities, you *will* be in-the-know for real to make real changes.

If you are not growing, you are dying.

Don't subscribe to being pompous and arrogant to the point you think that you can not receive valuable information from outside of yourself. It has been often said that you can learn even from children that have little to no experience in life. You know - *out of the mouths of babes.* You never know in what form life-saving information can come in so don't knock it until you try it!

Speaking on the subject of children, we as adults once marveled at the energy levels of children of how they fly around non stop. Or maybe you wondered before why children didn't need deodorants and perfumes. It is because they haven't had 20 or 30 years to pollute and contaminate there bodies with unhealthy foods that rot inside them and suck up their energy levels.

Who of you believe that you are healthy already? If you claim to be healthy, you probably still experience what people who think they already KNOW have and consider to be *normal* symptoms.

How about an occasional or recurrent headache, dry mouth, bad breath, colds, heartburn, dandruff, skin rashes, daily aches and pains? These occasional medical conditions are not normal at all. The conventional medical establishment will have you think that they are normal ailments, then inevitably offer some cover-up-method to distract you. On the contrary, a truly healthy body does not have those symptoms that signal an unbalanced body where disease is crouching at the doorstep undiagnosed.

In reality, if you attracted this book into your life conceivably, you could be overweight, underweight, sick and/or borderline sick. You have read the statistics about how many of us don't even know we have been stricken with some sort of chronic disease until the last minute. For the rest, we just drop dead suddenly. Most of us within our community and otherwise don't even know what being truly healthy feels like because sickness has become our identity. Still, there are others that are not really concerned with being healthy, so they settle for mediocrity and say idiotic things like, "we all gotta die someday from something".

In comment to those, does it have to be sooner than later?

Do you have to slowly rot while getting to that inevitable day and miss out on precious moments with loved ones? Since death is the ultimate enemy of us all it would be much better to keep our enemy in front of us where we can see it with our mind's eye, have a measure of control how close we catch up to it as supposed to having it sneak up on us and overtaking us unawares and prematurely.

Recognize even the slightest discomfort from within and be diligent about getting to the root cause of it!

Step 2 - Clarity

Clarity is the second step to the corrective thought processes on the journey to wellness. Clarity leads to power. We should endeavor to achieve personal empowerment. Power translates as the ability to DO or ACT. The essence of healing and rejuvenating oneself involves having a choice, then doing and acting accordingly. You have a choice to believe the medical doctors, believe the government, food industry, diet industry, your friends and family - who know not more than you, or to believe in your body's own innate ability.

Clarify your *why. Why* do you want to lose weight? Is it just for the bomb red dress you wanna get into? Is it to impress that fly honey down the street that you want to take out?

How about making the decision to release excess weight from your body, so you can be as healthy and energetic and emotionally stable than ever before? How about because you have a wonderful family that you want to be around to see go to college, marry and have a family themselves?

Get real clear on why you want wellness for the long term. While nothing is wrong with wanting to do it for the lesser important reasons, again the goal is to shift to a higher level of consciousness and recognizing that line of thought would be short term thinking and it will not last long. When the going gets tough, do you think that they are strong enough reasons to persist? More than likely – not!

So make a mental note to self: *The bigger the "why", the easier the "how".*

When you can work through and correct your thinking, then and only then will you be ready to fully embrace new concepts to help you take control over your health and well being. You gotta get crystal clear on it - total clarity. Once you have that clarity, then you are moved to act. Action thus becomes the vehicle used to get you what you want. Use your figurative peripheral vision to spot potential potholes or roadblocks - what usually holds people back is fear.

Fear can be described as the anticipation of pain. We won't go into a long dissertation to understand that our culture has undeniably suffered excruciating pain in the past and even in the perfect present on many different levels.

Yes, we have been hoodwinked, bamboozled and you know the rest. If you don't, you can get a history lesson online at BlackHistory. com.

In any case, it has caused us to be very skeptical and doubtful of everyone - everything, real or imagined. Thus, we never take action. Too many of us are not living our dreams because of living our fears.

Fear keeps our men toted as the, "forgotten population" from going to the doctors and being discriminated against.

Fear keeps us from going in and not wanting to get an unhealthy diagnosis.

Fear stops our Black women from taking time out for themselves thinking that we will somehow be neglecting everyone else, the kids, the hubby, Big Mama.

Fear that if I try to lose weight, I might get on a scale and it says I haven't lost any weight, then what.

Fear that you cannot get completely free from the enslavement of unhealthy food cravings.

Fear that making healthy lifestyle changes would be too difficult and you won't be able to enjoy life or handle stress.

The response to all of the above is: What if Martin Luther King allowed his fear of persecution to stop him, or Malcolm X or Rosa Parks of hers?

Don't allow fear to keep you from experiencing the omnipotent, divine health everyone of us has the potential for. Know that you may have fear, but don't let it stop you. Most assuredly, don't deny that you have it. Be aware that if you haven't acted to change your current situation, fear is somewhere in the equation.

Our minds are naturally on the lookout for what *could* go wrong in a given situation with the unknown. It sounds something like: "What if I start a new healthy way of living? What if I can't maintain it? What if I fall off the wagon and start eating crazy again? Those herbs are not FDA approved, I might get sicker. I read something somewhere that said that natural stuff doesn't work as well as pharmaceuticals. How do you know if organic really is best, because it is so expensive to eat organic, I don't know!!"

Mark twain stated, "I *have had thousands of problems, most of which never happened.*"

Fear has taken up room and board in our heads with three roommates - ignorance, doubt and negativity. The lease has expired, and they all must find another collective mind and community to live in.

They no longer have a place in the Black community!

If you are rock solid on the awareness and clarity corrective thought processes; unhealthy, destructive habits are a thing of the past

If you are committed to personal growth in these areas so as to work on yourself daily, you are indeed ready to receive the key to what we have been waiting a lifetime for.

You are ready to find out what it is that has the propensity to change the very fabric of the African American people as never before.

You are in fact ready to embrace and accept the one and only true answer to our health crisis.

Take a deep breath and relax your mind for a moment - long enough to read a short story about what's going on within our bodies and ultimately why what has been missing is really the key to unlocking the mystery of optimal health for all!

Toxic Factory

Liken your body to a factory with your organs being co-workers working within your body. Each has very specific tasks to make everything in the factory run smoothly. This is just one scenario of things that can go awry in the factory (the body). Whenever the blood in your body has to work overtime from fighting off toxins, the liver (the man in charge) has to pick up the overload. Your liver already has about 500 different job assignments to do for the body and now has to triple his workload on account of managing and handling toxic waste from the large intestine.

With the liver having to work harder than a field slave as a result of poisoning, it will look to the colon (large intestine) for help. The colon's job is to handle taking out the trash (waste). However, the colon can't do its job properly because the owner of the factory (body) takes so many pills on top of eating garbage foods. With tons of sugary, salty, processed, fried, chemical-laden food flooding in all the time, there is a build-up of pounds upon pounds of toxic fecal matter that is glued to its walls. As a result the colon has lost its figure, is out of shape with no more muscle tone. The stress has literally taken its toll.

Since the liver is a loyal worker and a great team player, he just continues to work overtime until he becomes completely wore out. Of course, the owner of the factory (body) by now starts to experience disease within the body. Some of the signals include: constipation, indigestion, light headedness, heart palpitations, bad breath, headaches, depression, etc. When things get to be unbearable and as last resort, the owner (of the body) goes to the doctor. The doctor tells the owner that nothing is wrong, that all tests are normal, and says, "If it will make you feel better, let me prescribe you something to ease the discomfort."

Now the liver has to play commando and has to process poisons from drugs along with other toxic rubbish that the out-of-shape, sluggish colon failed to dispose of. The liver's back is up against the wall and has no choice but to lean on the kidneys for help. The kidneys act as the master chemists. As the chemists, their function is to help control the mineral content of your blood along with its acidity and pressure. They convert vitamin D to an active form necessary for proper bone development, and produce the hormone erythropoietin, which stimulates red blood cell production in your bones. You can not find better chemistry at work than what these guys do.

Did you know that the two kidneys filter the water in your blood? That's about five quarts in an adult - every 45 minutes! Under normal circumstances (healthy state), it would be all-in-a days work, but in this scenario, the kidneys aren't happy at all about having to take on O.O.P. (Other Organs Problems). The kidneys have been feeling the extra pressure for the past few years, due to the colon not showing up for work.

This snowball effect is overwhelming for the kidneys because they were not trained to handle weighty bowel toxins; Their job is to purify body fluids - like the blood. They are puzzled as to where all these toxins are coming from.

They intuitively know that these are not toxins from normal chemical processes, but rather toxins from waste and chemicals that made their way up from the large intestine. They just floated right back into the body's system.

 The liver starts to protest and advises the kidneys to approach the colon. With this advice, the kidneys finally muster up enough courage to approach the colon. However, they find no luck. At this point the colon has already clocked out. The kidneys keep working doing the best they can - with what they have. However as time passes, the first sign that the factory is about to fold is that: unruly, unwelcome guest referred to as "toxins" have entered the building. There are so many un-invited guests that the internal environment has gotten overly crowded; hotter and sweatier than a late-night house party.

The following symptoms begin to manifest like the ones mentioned earlier construed to be "*normal*":

✓ Mental fogginess

✓ Aches and pains

✓ Infections

✓ Digestive disorders

Until now, most of this toxic concoction has been shouldered by the kidneys. Being boxed in, now the kidneys have no where else to go but to the bladder. If you are familiar with the anatomy, you can just picture where the bladder is situated; just in front of the last part of the large intestine known as the *sigmoid colon.*

It is important to note that the tissues of the bladder don't get off clear and free either. It too has been held hostage! Since it is the closest organs to the colon; the colon has now spilled over its toxic waste into the bladder along with other organs. None of the organs are immune to this state of toxicity. Other effected organs would include ovaries, uterus and prostate. You can imagine how pressured they feel (literally).

In some people, this degradation of the company could manifest in different ways.

The story can go on and into many different directions with this type of domino effect: First the toxic colon, then the blood, liver, kidneys, bladder and commonly overlooked lymph system.

Speaking of which, the lymph system is crucial for good immune function. With no good immune defense, disease will reign supreme like a wreck-less governmental tyrant over the body. When all systems malfunction, we experience pain as the way of the body saying "Too much!" It is a cry for help and you do well to tune into.

One big no-no is for you to ignore your body's many pleas for help and allow the doctors to commence to slicing and dicing on your body parts. Even worse is to let them dope you up with drugs that don't do anything for you except harm your internal organs.

Stop overworking your organs and underpaying them! They will go postal on you!

Please understand that when the body reaches a peak state of toxic overload, it will retain water to dilute the poison. This is why people often can look swollen and/or feel puffy like a Goodyear blimp.

Not to mention the negative impact on the skin, but as the basis of this whole discussion, the factory (body) - will manufacture FAT.

The body, being very resourceful and equipped with built-in defense mechanisms, will have the organs huddle together to communicate. They all will encase themselves in fat and mucous; struggling to dodge the inevitable – cellular degeneration (perfect setting for cancer), organ failure and if unchecked - death.

All informed, qualified health professionals who have an ounce of integrity about them should be taking the time to educate their patients about this! If they don't or they won't, you should stay ahead of the learning curve so you may be fully informed.

You can exercise all you want, and you should because it's good for you, but if you expect to prevent disease and/or reverse it, you must give your body what it needs to do so. We must support our bodies internally.

If this is accomplished, it is nothing short of a miracle when you feel your body responding favorably from being fed nutritionally. Then, you start to see a healthy glow about yourself, and start to see tonality and have a nice lean posture.

Now, it's time to discuss the missing links to create this miracle.

III.

SOLUTIONS TO REVOLUTIONIZE YOUR OVERALL HEALTH

My Personal Health Statement:

I am committed to…

_____

I am committed because…

1) _____

2) _____

3) _____

4) _____

5) _____

My potential obstacles are…

1) _____

2) _____

3) _____

4) _____

5) _____

My weaknesses are…

1) _____

2) _____

3) _____

4) _____

5) _____

Be aware of them, so you can work on them daily!

My strengths are…

1) _____

2) _____

3) _____

4) _____

5) _____

Hone your strengths to manage around your weaknesses!

My short-term health goals are... (1-2 yrs from today)

1) _____

2) _____

3) _____

4) _____

5) _____

My long-term health goals are... (3-4 yrs from today)

1) _____

2) _____

3) _____

4) _____

5) _____

I plan to achieve these goals by ____/____/_____

"BELIEVE AND ACT AS IF IT WERE IMPOSSIBLE TO FAIL!"
– Charles Kettering

"I Stand"

By Damon Reed

Family, Friends, Allies, Foes, Believers, Doubters, Ladies and Gentlemen, I stand before you today a success of yet another life changing endeavor. I stand before you as a testimonial memorial of perseverance, dedication, and devotion. I stand triumphant over the raging rivers of life. Beaten and bullied by the waves of failure, yet here I stand! Often slammed against the rocks of slander on the shores of envy, but kept on track by the encouraging voice of The Most High. At times I was drenched by the rains of self-doubt and I found myself staring down the barrel of digression, but a preserved wisdom would rise to regenerate my self-belief and renew my decomposing self-image so still I stand. I once stood as a scapegoat of the shortcomings of my peers and accused of drowning in the sea of passivity, but those that cross bridges that will never be built are doomed to drown in the saliva that fell from their mouths as they anticipated my failures. Due to my gender and skin tone I have been presumed incompetent by the unrelenting gestures of America. But led by the spirits of my ancestral predecessors I have escaped the traps of that stereotypical predestined path and so I stand as an example and not a statistic. Although debilitating and grinding adversity would amplify my struggles and attempt to chain me to the lowest rung of the economic ladder, the encouraging words of a loving mother and the supporting presence of friends and family would allow me to demonstrate an overcoming characteristic genetically implanted by those that stood where I now stand. My recent accomplishments are but a fragment of the test of times. There will come a day when again I would be faced with depleted self-confidence. Again I will be reclined in the path of adversity. Another time will come when I am exhausted by the blows of injustice. I will have to endure the storms of a system designed for my annihilation again and again. And I will again be standing in the fires of slander and ridicule. Oh but when the smoke clears I will be seen standing with my feet planted firmly against the Earth's crust and knees strengthened by my will to go on and my head lifted to receive further guidance from God Almighty. I will be seen STANDING! I stand, as a product of the Kings and Queens of Great Africa. I stand, for the unyielding inspiration of little black girls and little black boys. I stand, in the doorway keeping the doors of opportunity from closing. I stand, for every man and every woman that said it couldn't be done. I stand, as an exception to the American rule. I stand, for the struggle endured by my slave ancestors. I stand, as my sister and brother's keeper. I stand, as a voice for the braided heads and sagging pants of the ghettos. I stand, as the potential of my incarcerated black men and black women. For equality, I stand. For justice, I stand. For righteousness, I stand. For truth, I stand. In the Name of the Heavenly Father, I stand. Victoriously, I-Stand!

Simple Weight Loss Tips and Suggestions

1 - Drink an 8 oz glass of (purified or distilled preferably) water first thing in the morning. This will initiate good body metabolism and cleansing.

2 - Eat your last meal of the day before 7pm. After this time, your body has to work too hard to break down and metabolize food.

3 - Take digestive enzymes (preferably live enzymes). Chances are, if you are overweight – you have problems with digestion and often experience constipation, and bloating. This is caused by your body not digesting food properly.

4 - Consume only organic meats, poultry, and fish. Organic meats and items do not contain preservatives, and are not injected with hormones and antibiotics. You can purchase these items at health food stores such as Trader Joe's, Wholefoods, and Wild Oats.

5 - Add live cultured foods to your diet. Organic yogurt and kefir, as well as unpasteurized sauerkraut, have active enzymes that nourish your cells. Live foods give off a good vibration for rejuvenation.

6 - Stay clear of non-organic milk. If you choose to consume dairy, GO ORGANIC only. Here is an interesting fact to consider about non-organic dairy: the diseased cows that the government gets their dairy supply from has a level of pus that is legally acceptable according to government regulations. Although a couple of hundred thousand cells per ounce exist, most of us would agree that we could do without the disgusting pus in our dairy! For more information, visit www.notmilk.com

7- Minimize your intake of coffee and other caffeine-based products. Caffeine activates the stress hormone cortisol that causes you to gain weight. It should gradually be eliminated ideally with only occasional consumption.

8 - Everyday drink enough water that equals half your body weight in ounces. Practice this as close to perfection as possible.

This will flush toxins from your fat cells, and is absolutely necessary to lose weight.

9 - Eliminate all refined sugars from your diet. This includes white flour, which pretty much will turn to paste in your stomach.

10 - Cleanse. This is the most important suggestion. If you want to shed weight safely, and keep it off - you must cleanse and detoxify your body. Once you rid yourself of toxins, the body will no longer need to manufacture fat to protect itself. No magic, no mystery - It just makes sense. For specific recommendations, visit <u>www. CleanseFormula.com</u>

If you would like to come away from diet pills, fad diets and if you are tired of the myths and conspiracies to keep you overweight, there is a way to freedom from these shackles.

These solutions are intrinsically holistic in nature. In combination with good nutrition, and light to moderate exercise – it is helping thousands of people who first and foremost care about their health. As a wonderful side benefit, they lose weight.

It's not even about any one particular product. It's about a system that works synergistically with the body, and lets your body be the miracle and the amazing creation it was intended to be. Again, it does not have to be complicated in order to work.

Take this thought away with you that the power to lose weight and keep it off is already within you. You only need to give your body what it needs to function optimally and naturally release fat from a cellular level. The choice is yours! The information you are reading can always be at your fingertips for easy reference. You don't have to memorize anything.

Don't allow doubt or fear or negativity to cloud your judgment. As of now you are "free". Just remove your shackles!!

Healthy Foods

Natural Appetite Suppressants

1 - Green leafy vegetables like cabbage. When you fill your stomach with these foods, you feel full and satisfied. This is accomplished by switching off the hunger signals in the brain, so you don't consume too many calories and overeat.

2 - Pickles. Only buy all natural pickles that don't contain artificial ingredients. These too keep you full and satisfied because they take up a considerable amount of space in your stomach. They are capable of tuning off your appetite cravings.

3 - Apples. These are great appetite suppressants because the bulky fibers fill you up while managing appetite hormones. Also, the actual act of chewing apples helps hunger cravings.

4 - Raw organic apple cider vinegar. If you take 1 tsp before each meal, it helps you to burn stored fat.

5 - Organic unrefined virgin coconut oil. By taking 1 tsp in the morning and 1 tsp in late afternoon, this will help food migrate through the digestive track quicker as well as stimulate the thyroid. This in turn helps you burn fat while you sleep. You want "unrefined", so that you get the maximum benefits of the healthy fats it contains.

6 - Hot peppers. All kinds of these little guys help to increase metabolism which means you will burn more fat, and get more energy in your body.

Proper Exercise

For African Americans, this is the least preferred method of permanent weight loss for a couple of reasons that will now be addressed. Part of the frustration is as a result of the myths associated with weight loss. It leaves much to be desired in terms of seeing real results from exercise. What are we speaking about?

In short, to create energy your body burns fat or it burns sugar (glucose), but it can't burn them both simultaneously.

When exercising, once you enter into the aerobic zone (70% or more of your max. heart rate), your body will stop burning fat and immediately begin to burn blood sugar - since blood sugar can be converted to energy much faster than fat.

Aerobic exercise will burn fat, but only *after* you have depleted or exhausted your available blood sugar. This process takes at least 20 to 30 minutes of being in the aerobic zone.

Thousands of overweight individuals are on fancy and expensive exercise equipment, pedaling and running, like they are really getting something done. The sad thing is they are not burning fat. If there exercise regimen is at least an hour, the first 30 minutes is expended by burning off blood sugar. After that you need another 30 minutes to burn any fat. So if you are only on the machine for 10 or 20 minutes, not much is being accomplished. Interestingly enough, various types of exercise equipment continue to break sales records, but there are still record-breaking obesity statistics. In your mind, does that make sense?

Are you ready for truth? You have probably heard it a million times - here is a million and one more. The truth is that walking is the best type of exercise for sustained-healthy weight loss. Walking burns fat. The elliptical machines are nice, but old- fashioned brisk walking is still hands down, bar-none the best option for most. Walking also builds lean muscle which "leeches" off the body's excess fat so-to-speak. So the recommendation is to walk daily while making sure to drink plenty of water. Then, you will transform your body into a healthy, lean, fat burning machine that's capable of burning fat 24 hours of the day.

Before you decide to embark on any exercise regimen, every African American needs to warm up mentally to ensure full proof success. We are a busy people and we need to make the most out of our time that we will buy out for exercise. "Nothing can be more discouraging than starting an exercise program and not getting the desired results from lack of good mental preparation," says Brian Bailey of Fit Tyme Productions – inventor and founder of the Mental Hurdle of Fitness program.

Recognizing the many pitfalls in fitness, Bailey designed this program for mental pre-workout readiness. Bailey is an American Council on exercise and personal training, as well as a U.S. Air Force physical training leader that understands what we as a people need mentally for fitness success. "We always hear the talk of exercising and physical activity, but what about getting motivated to start," Bailey says.

Only after you move closer to your ideal weight, should you add some aerobic exercise and definitely moderate strength training. This can be beneficial as a great way to maintain your weight and support your heart, lung, muscles, and circulatory system.

Jumping on a trampoline is a proven asset to rejuvenating all of the cells in your body, as this increases good flow of oxygen. After all, you're only as healthy as your weakest cell. Trampolines provide more overall benefits for the body and are less expensive than a lot of exercise machines and gadgets. What ever you do, make sure you are sweating - as this will help to release stored toxins and naturally encourage weight loss.

Getting The Most Out Of Your Supplements and Vitamins

Are you daily supplementing your diet with a multi-vitamin pill or herbs of some kind? You should, in fact, be doing so already, but this key statement must be interjected before getting into the specifics:

You can take the best herbs, multi-vitamins, the best super juice tonic, and eat all the fruit and veggies you want. While these all are helpful, please understand that you will never get the maximum benefit from any of those regimens if you don't cleanse out the impurities from your body beforehand.

The old toxic waste material that is sitting inside our bodies rotting gives a home to mutant invaders. These invaders are worms, viruses, bad bacteria and fungus that live off of any vitamins we may take. If they are not CLEANSED first, your body cannot fully absorb what you are giving it.

With that being said, it is indisputable that in order to have a healthy body, we as humans are dependent on proper nutrition that must be supplied everyday of our lives. Sadly though, the Standard American Diet (SAD) is severely deficient in minerals, and the soil in which we depend on for our food source has been depleted of vital nutrients.

The United States Senate document #264 states: "Our physical well-being is more directly dependent upon the minerals we take into our systems, than upon calories or vitamins, or upon the precise proportions of starch, protein or carbohydrates we consume." Because American produce is now grown in highly depleted soil, even people who are cautious about what they eat simply can't get all the necessary nutrients. The alarming fact is that the foods, fruits, vegetables and grains that are now being raised, no longer contain enough of certain needed minerals.

As you can see, a very big challenge has been how to get the proper nutrition from what we eat, thus supplementation is no longer optional. Dr. Jean Mayer, a Harvard Graduate of Nutrition, states that many people need additional supplies of vitamins and trace minerals. Out the door goes the theory that all you need to do is "eat healthy foods" because basic understanding of that statement dictates that we don't get all the required nutrients from food. We need an outside source of vitamins and minerals.

Many people also still don't realize that without minerals, vitamins have no function. Having a marked or even a marginal deficiency in any one of the more important minerals could spell disease for us. What we have surmised is that thereafter, people will often turn to drugs and surgery because of lack of understanding that the root cause of their ailments may very well be from specific mineral or nutritional deficiencies.

Things have gotten so bad that even the American Medical Association is recommending that we all, at the very least, should be taking a multi-vitamin pill.

An additional point of interest for African American women who are concerned about having strong, long healthy hair should definitely be supplementing their diets with vitamins and minerals. When you already have a deficiency of vitamins and nutrients in the body, it will compensate by pulling nutrients from the hair, skin and nails to go to support more vital organs and body functions to survive. After all, you can still live and be relatively healthy without nutrients for hair, skin and nails. But you know how meticulous Black women are about their hair!

African American men pride themselves in handling their business behind closed doors. However, of late there are a great number of them experiencing low levels of testosterone. This leads to decreased stamina, strength, endurance, less strong erections or maintenance of erection. All of these symptoms can easily be corrected and satisfied with appropriate and specific vitamin and mineral supplementation. No, we are not talking about Viagra or any other drug featured in those 3am infomercials! Rather, we are talking about high quality nutritional herbs.

Many of us do care about our overall health and want to experience health bliss, but are at a lost when it comes to purchasing potent, but safe health supplements. We feel that if we are going to spend money supplementing our diets, we want to make sure that we get the full benefits of the nutrients.

Notwithstanding, price doesn't necessarily equal quality.

There is a quick, full proof test to determine what you are really getting in your health supplements. Just remember that no matter how much you spend, if the supplement is not absorbable - you're just throwing away your money because you're not receiving the full benefit of the product. These must be identified because we don't want everyone making a marathon dash for GNC, thinking that they are going to be getting quality because it's the most recognized name brand chain of stores.

So, how should one gauge the effectiveness of health supplements?

Tablet Vitamin Supplements

If you have tablet vitamins in your cabinet, when you take them you're only getting about 10-15% absorption. So hypothetically, if you spend $100 on vitamins you will have wasted $90.

There are two reasons for this minimal absorption:

1) Tablets are made up of a lot of "extras" that are foreign to the body like: toxic binders, fillers, glues, and coatings - all of which can actually stifle the body's efforts to absorb nutrients.

2) A lot of these pills have a highly metallic-count which will make your body work really hard to try and digest substances that have a consistency of pebbles or stones.

What these companies will do in most cases is add massive doses of nutrients, that when consumed, cause much stress on the kidneys and the liver. We already have learned how important those organs are to us, not to mention the fact that all these ingredients are then smashed into a tablet by heat and pressure, further damaging and degrading nutrients by another 25%.

Capsule Vitamin Supplements

If you have capsule vitamins, you will get about 30-50% more than that of tablets. This is the next best thing if you can't get liquid vitamins. Since the nutrients are maintained in their original form; they won't have the same level of toxicity as that of tablets.

Liquid Vitamin Supplements

Liquid vitamins and minerals are the superior choice of vitamin supplementation. Nothing needs to be broken down for the body to absorb. They can get into the bloodstream more efficiently. However, not all liquid vitamins are the same. For process of elimination, here are some questions to ask:

- Are the ingredients organic?

- Do they contain live enzymes?

- How bio-available (easily absorbed) are they?

- Are the dosages of nutrients balanced - and if so how they are processed?

- Did the manufacturer have the right level of expertise to balance the nutrients out?

In addition, you must find out if the company or individual(s) is reputable.

Conceivably, if you select the right liquid vitamin and mineral supplement the absorption rate could be close to 100%.

This is not a complete list, but it is a basis to start out with. At minimum, this information should cause you to realize the importance of proper nutrition and the need to be selective in choosing a clean source of supplementation!

Internal Cleansing

Internal cleansing is your very own secret weapon to cope with things that plague and rob each of us of good health and vitality. Building blocks to good health have been given in a systematic manner, and now it's time to gain momentum to get you to the ultimate destination; quickly, safely and most of all-naturally!

Make no mistake about it: you must be regularly cleansing your body of toxic substances present in the food we eat, the air we breathe, the water we drink - as well as nutritionally supporting it. You are fooling yourself, if you think that you will otherwise achieve pristine health and/or address sustained weight loss. To put it another way: You are sorely mistaken if you think that you can continue to eat poisonous foods, take prescription drugs and not be adversely affected. Internal cleansing can help lessen the damaging effects to your current health, promote anti-aging and as a wonderful side benefit – release stored fat!

Just like any other product or service, there are hundreds of different types of cleansing methods available now in health food stores and on the Internet, but all are not created equal. Some even require administration by a licensed health professional. While all types are certainly superior and safer than drugs and surgery, you can choose from the good, the better, and the best.

Please believe, in the world as we know it today, that optimal health is neither achievable nor sustainable through any other method other than - nutritional cleansing. It is very necessary to be redundant about this point!

Here are some of the most popular ones:

- **Fasting** is a form of cleansing that you can do yourself, where you will be omitting solid foods for a time and consuming only liquids so your body's energy can concentrate on ridding itself of toxins and allowing rest for internal organs. Fasting for extended periods of times are generally not recommended for any reason. Generally, a 24-48 hour cleanse is very safe and extremely effective. This provides for excellent spiritual, emotional, and physical harmony!

- **Hyperthermia** is a form of cleansing where you artificially create fever within your body to boost immune function. This is very effective for eliminating toxins and infectious bacteria, due to bacteria being unable to survive in high temperatures. This can be done in a sauna at the gym or in a spa with infra-red sauna beds.

- **Ionic Foot Detox** is a form of cleansing where toxins are drawn out of the body thru the pores of the feet by a group of atoms carrying a positive or negative charge. This is as a result of gaining or losing one or more electrons called an ion. This effects whether or not the body will remain in a healthy state. These ions will charge, energize and rebalance the cells within your body and help release toxins in the water. Most experience immediate results. This is usually administered in your local spa, chiropractic office or natural health practitioner's office. You may purchase the equipment online as well.

- **Juice Therapy** is the process of only consuming fruit juices extracted from actual fruits. Organic fruits are highly recommended. These can enhance cleansing and detoxification when used as part of a tailored health maintenance plan. One great daily juice combination is fresh celery, apple and carrot juice.

- **Colon Hydrotherapy** is a form of cleansing, where you get a series of deep colonic water flushes to detoxify the colon to remove old built-up waste. This helps to improve digestion! Also known as colonics, these sessions are usually administered by a licensed colon hydro-therapist. Consult with him/her to determine the necessary amount of sessions.

- **Lymphatic Drainage** helps accelerate the flow of lymph fluids and drainage pattern used throughout the body. The lymph system detoxifies your organs that are frequently overlooked. This is usually administered by a licensed natural health practitioner or can be given manually by a certified massage therapist.

- **Hydrogen Peroxide Therapy** is a form of cleansing where hydrogen peroxide is administered by a licensed natural health care practitioner intravenously. This is useful in ridding the body of toxins very quickly and is an effective alternative to treating viral infections, Candida (yeast overgrowth), acne and more! There is a hospital in Mexico that has a 100% success rate in treating cancer in just a matter of weeks by giving intravenous ozone and hydrogen peroxide. Simply go online, and research how you can get more information to utilize it.

- **Oxygen Therapy** is similar to hydrogen peroxide therapy, but oxygen therapy is a form of cleansing that is introduced orally, transdermally or infused. It is able to rid the body of toxicity, bacteria, and parasites. It is also used as a powerful alternative healing treatment for serious illnesses such as cancer. From a scientific standpoint, cancer and viruses cannot survive in an oxygen-rich environment.

- **Chelation Therapy** is a form of cleansing that uses specific high-grade minerals, especially designed to bind with chemicals and toxic materials. This draws them out of the body safely and effectively, and can be accomplished by

I.V. as well. It is a powerful treatment for arteriosclerosis and arterial plaque - both complications associated with heart disease. It is found to be beneficial for treatment of ADHD, lupus and more

- **Skin Brushing** helps the skin to directly eliminate waste acids. The skin is one of the main and largest organs to detoxify as the body makes new skin every 24 hours. So skin brushing keeps the uppermost layer free of dead skin cells that can slow down oxygen absorption throughout the body. This can be done at home using a natural bristle brush only in the shower with brisk, upward movements. You should brush with enough vigor and just enough pressure to create a slight flush-tint to the skin. This too does not represent all available cleansing plans, but is a wonderful list for the beginner.

Other cleanses include Candida cleanse, kidney cleanse, and liver & gallbladder cleanse. Some cleanses can be done yourself, and others must be done by licensed health experts. The current condition of your health will determine which form you might choose. For more specifics or recommendations, visit www.cleanseformula.com

Since everyone's state of health can vary widely, it is realistic to expect and respect the fact that certain changes will take place when you cleanse. Some of our experiences will differ. Therefore, enhancing your body's chemistry to one that supports health longevity is of utmost importance. When you choose to embark upon the process of utilizing any type of cleansing regimen, you should prepare to encounter certain reactions. What are they?

What to Expect From Cleansing

When healing is taking place, some may think they are having a 'bad reaction' to a cleansing. This is just a natural occurrence that the body may experience as it tries to move upwards to reach it's destination of better health; shifting gears to better nutrition.

Once this happens, some of the time (not all) people may experience minor discomfort of some nature. Initially, one may feel a euphoric like or a natural high. Understand whenever we improve on what we put (or don't put) into our bodies, it becomes better at "cleaning house" and changes will occur.

Another possibility is that sometimes the symptoms of past disorders may re-occur as a result from cleansing. This is on account of the body's natural process of healing itself from the head-down and from the inside-out. Natural health professionals commonly reference these effects as "tissue memory", whereas an organism has the ability to store, recall and retain the memory of past symptoms or imbalances.

This tissue memory may be released during the cleansing process. But remember this point:

It's unnecessary to try to fight against it, simply go with the flow. It is vital that we re-experience past symptoms in a positive manner. Positive feelings include grace, love, forgiveness, and most importantly - non-resistance. These are all supportive and nurturing in this delicate process! Forgiving those who have hurt you is also *key* since resentment actually makes you toxic.

The science of quantum physics point to and shows that the body is a product of our thoughts. So if you have negative thoughts and feelings, it will only perpetuate sickness within. On the other hand, thoughts or feelings of gratitude, love and the like essentially lead to a happier, healthier biochemistry. This is the reason the greatest book ever written mentions that a calm heart makes one happy. We will talk more about that book later.

Uncomfortable symptoms are always short in duration and before you know it you will be riding the freedom train of heavenly bliss!

For the sake of discussion, let us just clarify what disease means - disease is any condition where the body is without ease (dis-ease). To that end, any given diseased state is three-fold: mental, emotional and physical - and there is simply no getting around this fact!

Some other rather innocent symptoms may include slight lethargy, or a mild headache. The good news is that these usually only last at most – 72 hours. Keep all of this in mind while cleansing, so as not to get confused and mistake the symptoms and feelings of healing as a "sickness" or a bad reaction.

You need to be patient, yet diligent during the healing process. When this is achieved, the payoff is immeasurable and results are incomparable. Hopefully, you have been convinced and fully accept that humans create disease by poisoning themselves slowly over time. It takes years to get out of balance. Cause for celebration is that it will not take years to correct. Mainstream society may argue till dooms day that certain diseases are incurable. Dr. John Demartini, a philosopher, says, "*Incurable* just means *curable* from within!" So keep that in mind every day of your cleansing, and you can and will be successful!

What else must one do to get the most out of their cleansing regime?

Pre-cleanse Instructions

- Seek out a pure water source for drinking, in order to consume at least half your body weight in ounces every day. Also, have a glass in the morning as soon as you awaken to jumpstart daily cleansing and metabolism.

- Change what you eat and where you eat. Shop at health food stores and farmer's markets. In many cases, when you buy foods that are in season they tend to be more affordable than foods sold at regular supermarkets.

- Clear the refrigerator and cabinets of all items not on your cleansing protocol and replace them with your favorite choice of organic fruits, raw veggies, whole grains (like brown rice), and healthy oils (flax oil, olive oil, and coconut oil). Flax oil can be used for weight loss, and helps you stay in the fat burning zone longer.

- Exercise and be consistent with your exercise regimen, but do switch it up sometimes to keep it interesting so your body won't stop making progress. You can walk, run, swim, or do any other thing mentioned in the previous exercise chapter. Most suggestions are not only invigorating, but also relaxing.

- Abstain from smoking, alcohol or caffeine while cleansing as these all suppress the immune system. It takes the body approximately 17 hours to neutralize the effects of caffeine. You may be pleasantly surprised that you are not as interested in those harmful substances, upon adding this lifestyle change.

- Plan ahead on which cleansing protocol(s) you want to incorporate in your new healthy lifestyle. Don't wait until the last minute. You want to be ready. Disregarding this advice can be catastrophic. Surely, you have heard the old adage: *Haste makes waste!*

- Mentally prepare by collecting and gathering all necessary items prior to your intended start date.

- So that you have total clarity (which is step 2 in the corrective thought processes that you have just learned), go over your cleansing plans. Be familiar with your goals, so that during the week before you start, friends or family can track your progress. Maybe they could even buddy up with you for additional support.

- Call to mind sources of inspiration and reminders of healthy living choices. Put them on your walls, desk at work, bathroom mirror, dashboard in your car, etc.

- Effectively manage stress. The body needs 100% of its energy to regenerate, recharge and heal itself. A phenomenal stress management system is the UCURE Power Break System. This happens to the best in technological advances and overall permanent results. Energetic rebalancing is useful too. Additional reasons to reduce stress include the fact that the muscles have difficulty repairing themselves when stress is present. Unresolved stress and poor diet are the root causes for alopecia - hair loss in Black women.

- Sleep. Staying up late can throw off your body's composition and suppress the natural sleep hormone Melatonin. Mainstream medicine agrees that your body can only repair and heal itself between 10pm and 2am.

- Take your PH-levels before and after a cleanse. This offers valuable information over the course of your cleanse. [To understand more about PH testing, see the box below]

About PH Testing

Similar to a thermometer reading, PH testing is a practical, easy and useful way to check your body's internal environment. You can gauge whether or not your body is functioning in a healthy state.

The optimal range is between 7.0 and 7.5. The moderate range is between 6.5 and 6.75. The unhealthy range is between 6.0 and 6.25. (If you have an unhealthy range, you must consider proper dietary changes.)

The dangerous range is between 4.5 and 5.75. (If you have the dangerous range, you must seek the assistance of a licensed professional.)

Here are some other tips and suggestions you may incorporate in your cleansing program:

- Each day, commit to sticking to the plan. If you're gonna hit, you gotta commit! Refer to the health commitment section of this book, and remind yourself daily about your goals.

- Keep a journal of your progress. Record any troubling thoughts and even foods that you have eaten.

- Stay hydrated. Water increases oxygen and nutrient absorption by 600% when cleansing. Consider adding an appropriate (non-toxic) electrolyte drink to your water.

- Get a massage and/or chiropractic adjustment. For the best massages that specifically incorporate cleansing methods, visit www.pampermeplease.net

- Get a colonic, or second choice - an enema

- Try dry skin brushing

- Do not freak out if you find it difficult to stop thinking about food. This is a symptom of withdrawal from harmful substances you've been eating for nearly a lifetime. Then too, the level of emotional charge surrounding eating foods is not always apparent to us. Don't be hard on yourself, rather reflect back on your commitment remaining focused to get the full benefit from your cleanse. Also, you may think that you are hungry, but in fact you could be thirsty.

- Always, always, always take digestive enzymes before or with every meal. (this depends on the brand)

- It also would be a good idea, the day before, to eat some raw or steamed veggies with a clean source of protein for lunch, and a large leafy green salad with even more veggies for dinner. You can't OD.

Now you're all set. Ready, go 'cleanse'!

Why Cleanse For Spiritual Health?

Spirituality and the African American community have long been the pillars that we depend on to keep us grounded in all areas of our lives. Now, due to the physical, emotional, mental, and financial despair we have had to contend with, the spiritual pillars that have been our foundation is now being shaken to its core.

Even as far back as slavery times, it was spirituality that kept the slaves going amidst troublesome times. Today, we are in equally troublesome times of our own. The very foundation that we once depended on, is not even there to be that support structure because they are in grave danger themselves.

This book could not be completed without covering multi-facets of problems that have arisen for Black folks to overcome, without giving the utmost attention to our rich heritage of spirituality. There must be a concerted effort and focus on the restoration of its leadership role.

If the spiritual leaders are still in fact leadership for the Black community, it must lead by example without doubt.

If we are too ill or too physically challenged, how can we in the community or those who believe in a higher-being worship wholeheartedly? How can we truly serve our fellow man to the full?

The most important commands are to love your God and your neighbor. How are we even capable of doing this to the greatest extent when we haven't loved ourselves enough – first?

We are not being loving to ourselves when we run our bodies down by being over-occupied with the cares of life and don't take ample time to replenish and properly nourish them.

Yes, even with those in the spiritual community, there are too many suffering from obesity with related illnesses - and you know who you are!

There have been so many lives claimed unnecessarily, including some of the greatest leaders that African Americans have depended on for support.

For those that remain, you are a walking example of what you believe. It is inconsistent to preach about godliness, cleanliness and appreciativeness for life that our creator has given us, when we are not doing so ourselves.

Don't we have a responsibility to our creator to take care of this gift? Thus the question: How are we taking care of this gift?

It's like someone very special to you giving you a gift, maybe a rare and beautiful vase or some other precious pottery. Would you allow someone to urinate in it and disrespect it in that manner? Of course not!

When we choose to put garbage into our bodies and then fail to clean it out properly, that is essentially what we are doing. The body is capable of handling the normal task of cleansing as it was naturally designed to do so, but as we have ascertained - it needs help, not hindrance.

So what we should be doing, each and every one of us from the leadership on down is cleansing our body, "temple".

We should do so regularly since the world that we live in is toxic and probably will continue to be. Most of us take the time every day to keep our outer bodies clean by bathing regularly, brushing our teeth, and so forth. African Americans in general tend to be very meticulous about clean, "fresh" clothing and well-kept hair. In fact, it's been said that Blacks are the sharpest people you will ever meet.

We take especially good care of the vehicles we drive through routine tune-ups and oil changes to keep them running smoothly and working well for us.

How much more so should we be doing that for the most precious gift of life that we have? Internal cleansing is the most effective, beneficial way that we can clean our bodies out to keep it running smoothly and from breaking down on us.

Not only that, cleansing has roots as far back as ancient times when the disciples would fast and offer up supplications as mentioned in the book of Luke. Also mentioned, is that King David was renewed after fasting; which is a form of cleansing. The book of Joel written way back in the ninth century says, "Sanctify a time of fasting".

The greatest man that ever lived, himself fasted for 40 days. Of course, we know that fasting is not mandatory for spirituality purposes anymore. Neither is it recommended or necessary for that length of time today. The point is that cleansing the body temple helps us physically, mentally, and emotionally - out of which springs spiritual benefits too.

For emphasis, we can not be most effective in our spiritual life if we don't have clarity, oneness of mind, and abundance of energy to fulfill our spiritual obligations. Cleansing unequivocally and effortlessly gives us joy!

If you don't trust the sources from which the information on the latter pages came from; you can trust scriptural principles! For in such lies the truth, the ONLY truth!

The Bible does not hold the record of bestselling book of all times for nothing; This book is not outdated in any shape form or fashion.

Had Christopher Columbus turned to this great book to answer questions about the earth, he would have known that the earth was round and not flat.

The information was there thousands of years before, he just didn't EXPLORE it!

Let that be a lesson for us all when we are trying to decipher information. The Bible has proven to be scientifically sound in teaching our ancestors sanitary guidelines to prevent disease that we are just now catching up to, but will never surpass.

The whole point of why we needed to write this publication has shown the world how not following scriptural advice has ultimately been our own demise.

For every thought conveyed here-in, represents a scriptural principle that was broken, ignored or done in excess and not moderation.

This even goes for the morality aspects of the world's governments and companies.

Thousands of years beforehand, we all were forewarned and cautioned about overeating, overdrinking, and defilements of the body (smoking) - which unquestionably defiles the internal organs.

No, it doesn't directly say "don't eat trash foods with chemicals and in excess, or even not to smoke", but the principle *is* there of not defiling the body.

It has now been uncovered for you how specific foods degrade vital organs and harm the body over time. We can begin to undo the damage by adhering to the bible's timeless principles.

Intellects and scholars, if you are truly leaders, you need to make this message a permanent part of your lesson to all who have an ear to hear with understanding.

If these insights resonate with you - great, and if not - great too! However, the greatest man that ever lived stated this, and this subject will end on this note, "My sheep will hear my voice and recognize it!"

It is truly amazing when you start to feel yourself becoming more spiritually-inclined. You actually feel like giving a 100% to every facet of your life. How wonderful would it be to experience THE Life?

T - Total

H - Health

E - Euphoria

Life

"In a fear inspiring way I am wonderfully made". - King David of Ancient Israel

Our body is a miracle, cleansing it acts a catalyst to help it be that to the fullest potential. Our inner world affects our outer world. So, if you gleam nothing else from this section, believe that cleanliness is next to godliness!

Nutritional Cleansing - The Missing Link!

It's been broken down to you why the current system for losing weight and keeping it off, has been a failure for us as Black people and the world in general. You have been taught the concept of cleansing that is age old, but nonetheless extremely effective at addressing our health concerns supported by factual and scriptural basis.

It has been pounded into your minds indelibly, the utmost importance of proper nutritional supplementation along with nutritional foods. Noteworthy right from the onset, we highlighted the various elements that serve to impede progress with our overall health. These included educating the Black people on how to get out of our own way!

In doing all of this, we have given everyone multiple choices and methods of cleansing techniques to choose from based on their individual needs and/or preferences. What we have waited a lifetime for though, is the one-two punch that can give us in one swoop what has been talked about throughout this book.

Congratulations you have waited very patiently!

There is not a more appropriate, nor perfect time than the present to officially introduce to the Black community, the revolutionary solution to overall wellness. Nutritional cleansing is the only common-sense approach that has the propensity to change the very health fabric for the African American people in this 21st century.

In this respect, nutritional cleansing is the ultimate solution to helping Blacks reclaim their throne to a higher health status and lose weight. This solution cleanses the body at the cellular level, while simultaneously flooding your body with top grade, high-quality nutrients. This is currently not found in any other foods or any other therapy program.

You have searched high and low, now you needn't search anymore. This is literally your complete "meal ticket". This is the answer most of us have waited a lifetime for to eradicate this beast-of-burden of obesity. Diets, pills, drugs, surgeries, injections, and fancy recipes have failed. Now it's time to succeed!

This book has revealed to you that obesity can not be addressed unless underlying imbalances have been satisfied. Toxicity creates imbalances; Cleansing fully and effectively addresses this.

Discover visually how and why nutritional cleansing works!

Traditional Diet vs. Cleansing Flow Chart

This flow chart shows why diets are not successful for long-term weight loss, as they do not address the need to cleanse the body of impurities.

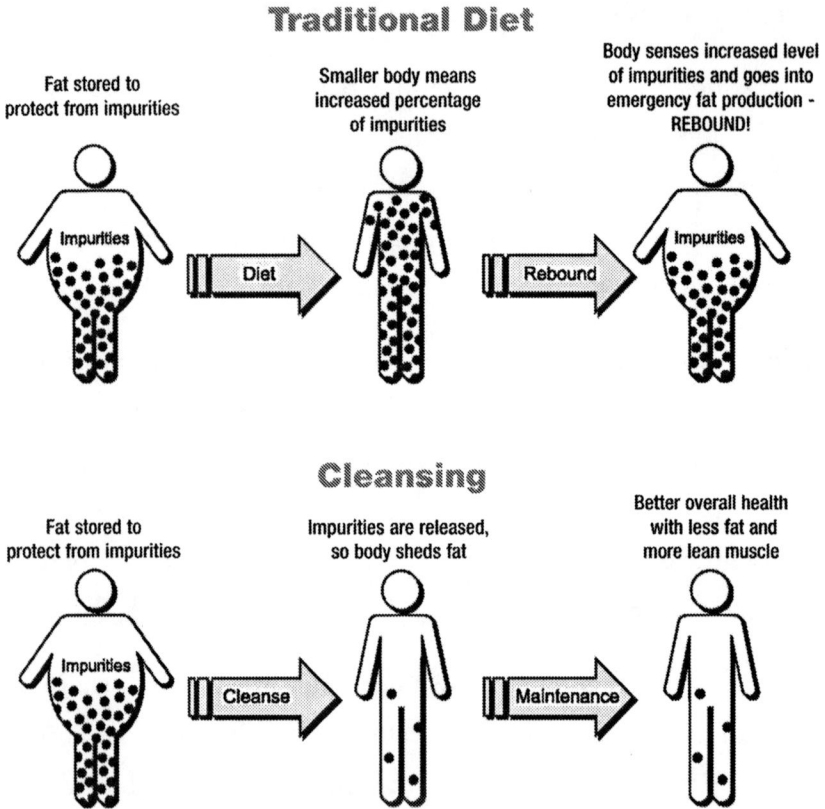

Traditional Diet

Fat stored to protect from impurities

Smaller body means increased percentage of impurities

Body senses increased level of impurities and goes into emergency fat production - REBOUND!

Impurities

Diet

Rebound

Impurities

Cleansing

Fat stored to protect from impurities

Impurities are released, so body sheds fat

Better overall health with less fat and more lean muscle

Impurities

Cleanse

Maintenance

Source: Isagenix International

144

Fad Diets vs. Cleansing and Replenishing

Fad Diets	Cleansing and Replenishing
Often nutrient deficient.	Give the body more nutrient-rich protein, carbs, fat and minerals.
Quick fix.	Is a long-term lifestyle approach to internal health.
Continued Cravings.	Balances brain chemistry to decrease cravings.
Nutritionally Restrictive.	Floods the body with high grade nutrients.
Focuses On Weight Loss.	Focuses on quality of life and longevity.
Does not enforce good eating habits.	Enforces great long-term nutritional habits.
Stresses the body.	Fuels the body.
Does not address cleansing the body.	Cleanses the body of toxins and impurities.

Source: Isagenix International

Here is a medical study summary to further support that nutritional cleansing is the only way to safe weight loss and optimal health:

MEDICAL STUDY:
The Effects of a New Food Technology on Body Composition, Body Systems And Blood Chemistries
Dennis Harper, DO
Thomas McNeilis, DO
Cynthia Watson, MD
Bryan Turner, DVM, MD

Abstract:

Obesity and its associated degenerative diseases including heart disease continue to rise in an unrelenting epidemic. Despite media attention to the magnitude of the problem, people continue in lifestyles that promote disease. However, a growing number in the population recognize the need for personal responsibility in health matters. A new food technology bringing a fresh approach to the problem has helped numerous individuals recapture many aspects of health including substantial weight loss. This cleansing system has captured the attention of the medical community as well because the results are gained without added stimulants, herbs or drugs.

An evaluation of the effects of the "nutritional cleansing"* was performed to systematically examine body composition as measured by deltoid skin-fold or impedance analysis.

Moreover, analysis of serum chemistries, lipids, and a comprehensive review of body systems were performed to identify subjective as well as objective findings associated with this technology.

This abstract, reprinted in its entirety, is intended to provide a balanced view of the available scientific information related to the Isagenix System This information is intended for general educational purposes and not to sell specific products. This does not constitute labeling, endorsements or advertisements for any particular products and should not be interpreted as recommending how to treat any particular diseases or health-related conditions.

Here are just a few of the many notables that have reaped rewards from nutritional cleansing and who want the world to know about it. The majority of the people who have made this healthy lifestyle change are average people who are sick and tired of being sick and tired.

Testimonials

"I really did get heavy, but I did a program....It's a weight program and it got me down. It's a huge difference for me. I'm flying around, I'm full of joy and energy." -- Roy Williams of the Dallas Cowboys

"I couldn't believe the superior benefits that I got from it. Immediately it started producing the brain chemistry of health, happiness and increasing romance - and this is what my field is all about..." -- John Gray PhD, author of *Men Are Mars, Women are From Venus*

"I've been so impressed with what [nutritional cleansing] has done for my life, the life of my family and the lives of my friends that I decided to write a chicken soup for the soul book...It's called Chicken Soup for the Healthy Soul, and it's comprised of stories of people's success..." -- Jack Canfield, co-author of *Chicken Soup for The Soul*

Here is what some from our very own community had to say:

"Two years ago I was experiencing a low ebb in my life. I was low mentally, physically and spiritually as well. Though I had been on a journey to improve my health, I was at a stand still. I was introduced to this wonderful program that promised to change my life, and I did it. Within hours of starting this program, I experienced increased energy unlike ever before, I began to think clearer...I dropped inches and pounds

in a very short time and my outlook on life was WONDERFUL…I can't imagine what my life would be like If I didn't have this change. I'm glad I don't have to find out!" -- R. Hebb, CMT

"I wasn't a believer and I wasn't convinced until I decided to try it. I just got tired of the pain…I was nervous and unsure if it would work…I no longer felt down anymore. I lost pounds just messing around with it…. -- D. Springs, business professional

"…it was the easiest thing I have ever tried. I managed in a very short while – about six weeks to drop 26 pounds. Yes it was incredible, easy, and effortless and just plain simple to use. I've never really been big, but when I lost the pounds I could see a major difference and so did everyone else around me. It actually shocked me what little effort it took. All I did really is walk 3-4 times a week and followed the easy menu ideas and before I knew it, I was super thin and super FINE… I encourage any everyone to give it a chance and just watch the weight come off!" -- D. Epps, School District Administrator

"I cleansed for 30 days. My mind and body are renewed. You cannot live life as it truly is to be lived without cleansing. My results were felt in every aspect of my life… I cleansed my body, but even more profound, I cleansed my soul!" – J. Williams, business professional

For more heartfelt testimonials and visuals, visit: www. weightlosshalloffame.net

A Final Note To Readers

It has often been said that reading and writing can affect life deeply - at most levels. You have read, I have written, thus through the power of communication, great things are achieved.

It is my desire that each and every one of you apply this knowledge, as it is only useful if you do apply it. Not only should *we* make use of this valuable, health-empowering information for ourselves, but we should keep the cycle of sharing going.

Sharing may add value to another life, as well as your own. The fact that you attracted this book into your life means something miraculous lies ahead for you, but you must get started to find out what.

Change your life TODAY, since tomorrow unforeseen occurrences befall us all.

For a list of my personal recommendations of nutritional cleansing programs, visit www.CleanseFormula.com

"Cleanse Your Body…and Perfect Your Health!"

REFERENCES

People:

Agatston, Arthur, M.D.

Bailey, Brian

Baughman, Fred A.

Blaylock, Russell, M.D.

Blumenthal, David, M.D.

Bronner, Yvonne

Canfield, Jack

Copeland, Karen, O.D.

Day, Loraaine, M.D.

Graham, David, M.D.

Hall-Trujillo, Kathryn

Mayer, Jean, Ph.D.

Olney, John, Ph.D.

Prosch, Gus, M.D.

Satcher, David, M.D.

Sturm, Roland

Thurber, James

Tsalaky, Teresa

Walker, David

Wheeler, Bill, Ph.D.

Williams, Roy

Organizations:

American Obesity Association

Center For Disease Control and Prevention

Center For Media and Democracy

Environmental Pressure Group

Food And Drug Administration (FDA)

Journal of The Medical Association

Books:

Cooper, Ann

Lunch Lessons: Changing The Way We Feed Our Children

Erb, John

The Slow Poisoning of America

Gray, John, Ph.D.

Mars & Venus, Diet and Exercise Solution

Nestle, Marion, Ph.D.

Food Politics

Roberts, H.J., M.D.

Aspertame (Nutrasweet) Is It Safe?

Obesity Society

United States Department of Agriculture

Washington Black Leadership Forum

Washington Journal of Health Affairs

Articles/Research Studies:

Abrams, Allen, Gray (1993)

Associated Press

British Medical Journal (2007) Lancet Study

Life Extensions Magazine, "Death By Medicine"

Harris Interactive for McNeil Consumer Specialty for Pharmaceuticals

Journal of National Cancer Institute (NCI)

Journal of Neurology

Journal of Toxicological Sciences

Mellman Group and Public Opinion

Strategies (2007)

New York Times (2005)

Organic Consumers Association

SEER Surveilance Epidemiology and End Results

The China Study, T. Campbell et al

Truth Publishing Inc.

Newstarget.com

Pure Hoodia Inc article (2005)

United States Senate Document #264

Web Sites:

www.adhdfraud.org

www.huntermillergroup.com

www.lapband.com

www.msgtruth.org

www.targetmarketnews.com

www.wholefoodfarmacy.com

RESOURCES

4girlsand1boy.wholefoodfarmacy.com

BlackDoctor.org

BlackNews.com

BodySculpt.org

BrianKBailey.com

CleanseFormula.com

Damon@superiorimagefitness.com

FreedomHealthSolutions.com

PamperMePlease.net

NaturalCures.com

RadiantGreens.com

UpRightFoods.com

About The Author

Makeisha Lee is a heavy researcher in the field of alternative health with her expertise focusing on detoxifying and cleansing the body. She is dedicated to research on a global scale and to delivering the most powerful, efficient, up-to-the minute health programs through her diverse affiliations in the healing arts.

She grew in Baltimore Maryland and received formal training at the Theocratic Ministry School. This unique educational program is attended by millions around the earth in upwards of 200 lands. This special education has also given her over 21 years of experience in communications, doing research, analytical/organizational skills and instruction in the arts of extemporaneous public speaking.

Lee later moved to southern California to receive extensive training in alternative health where she worked very closely with Licensed Natural Health practitioners. Currently, she works with a whole team of health professionals.

She writes weekly columns for BlackNews.com, BlackDoctor.org, and hundreds of African American newspapers nationwide. She also appears regularly as a guest on urban radio stations. In addition, she has authored several publications including the *African American Guide to Cleansing* and the soon-to-be-released *The Real Life Huxtables*.

Some of Lee's business partners include high profile health professionals and authors such as Dr. Bill Wheeler - White House staff nutritional advisor to former presidents and various athletes; John Andersen - one of the top formulators in the world; and authors Dr. John Gray PhD (Men Are from Mars, Women Are from Venus) and Jack Canfield (Chicken Soup for The Soul). She travels all over the country and abroad speaking on a wide range of health topics, as well as teaching the African American community how to create wealth from investing in their health. She has already helped thousands realize and accomplish their goals.

Lee is a mother of five children and a wife to husband Dante Lee, who is the president and CEO of Diversity City Media. She is very passionate and dedicated to helping and sharing life-saving information with others to help free themselves from needless pain and suffering - whether physical or emotional. She feels a moral obligation to service humanity by helping them live happier, healthier and joyful lives.

Printed in the United States
100140LV00008B/1-75/A

9 781434 347381